SEVEN USES

FOR **50** ESSENTIAL OILS

Dr. Josh Axe
Jordan Rubin
Ty Bollinger

ISBN-13: 978-0-7684-5495-6

ISBN-13 eBook: 978-0-7684-5496-3

Printed in the USA

1 2 3 4 5 6 / 24 23 22 21

CONTENTS

GENERAL SAFETY & COMMON SENSE GUIDELINES

Here are some important safety recommendations that apply to the use of all essential oils. Read this list carefully—and then go enjoy your oils!

▸ When it comes to essential oils, a little goes a long way. Start with one to two drops and assess your tolerance and desired results before increasing amount.

▸ Many oils can be applied NEAT (undiluted, or without a carrier oil), but check each oil first to ensure it is safe to do so. When in doubt, dilute.

▸ Stop use immediately if irritation occurs.

▸ **Some oils are not safe to take internally.** Check the warnings for each oil before ingesting and only consume essential oils that are certified organic and labeled as dietary supplements.

▸ **Some essential oils are not safe to use while pregnant.** Check the warnings for each oil before use during pregnancy.

- ► If you are prone to mouth or throat irritation, put essential oils into a capsule or dilute it with a carrier oil or food (honey, applesauce, etc.) before swallowing.

- ► When adding essential oils to food or liquid, start with one drop and taste before adding more.

- ► Most essential oils should be taken with food and not on an empty stomach.

- ► Talk to your healthcare practitioner before using essential oils if you are taking any prescription medications, as some oils may have interactions when taken along with certain drugs.

- ► Do not use essential oils in the eyes or in the ear canals.

- ► Only use certified organic oils to ensure highest quality and purity—and to ensure safety for use on or in your body.

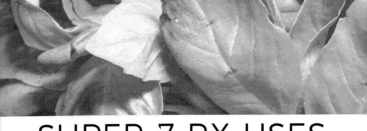

SUPER 7 RX USES
BASIL

1. Acts as an Anti-bacterial and Anti-fungal Agent

To combat bacteria and fungus in and around the home, diffuse or vaporize basil oil, or combine it with a natural cleaner in a spray bottle to rub down surfaces and help remove bacteria from kitchens and bathrooms.

2. Relieves Cold and Flu Symptoms

Diffuse basil throughout the home to fight common cold and flu symptoms such as congestion. Add 2 to 3 drops to a steam bath, or combine 2 drops of basil oil with 2 drops of eucalyptus oil and a carrier oil to help open up the nasal passages.

3. Freshens the Air

Aid in eliminating odor-causing bacteria and mold by diffusing basil oil, combining 4 to 6 drops with baking soda to clean kitchen appliances or spraying a mixture of water or natural cleaner and a few drops of basil oil in the toilet, shower and garbage can.

4. Aids in the Treatment of Urinary Tract Infections

Add 1 to 2 drops of basil oil to food, or dilute 1 to 2 drops with a carrier oil and take it internally to assist in detoxifying the urinary and digestive tracts.

5. Relaxes Muscles

Rub 3 drops of basil oil into painful, swollen muscles or joints to help relax them. To lessen tense areas and feel immediate relief, add Epsom salts, lavender oil and basil oil to warm bath water.

6. Reduces Ear Infection Discomfort

Rub equal parts basil and frankincense oil diluted with coconut oil behind the ears to help reduce swelling from an ear infection and encourage healing.[1]

7. Promotes Oral Health

Add a few drops of pure basil oil to your mouthwash or toothpaste. This will also help protect your teeth and gums from toothaches, ulcers, sores and viral blisters.

1.   Kristinsson, K.G., Magnusdottir, A.B., Petersen, H., Hermansson, A. (2005, January 12). Effective Treatment of Experimental Acute Otitis Media by Application of Volatile Fluids into the Ear Canal. *Infectious Diseases Society of America*. Retrieved from http://jid.oxfordjournals.org/content/191/11/1876.full

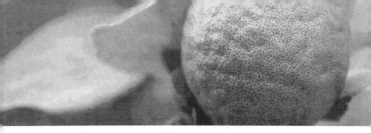

SUPER 7 RX USES
BERGAMOT

1. Improves Mood and Serves as a Natural Anti-depressant

Bergamot can create feelings of joy, refreshment and energy by supporting healthy circulation. Rub 2 to 3 drops onto your hands and cup your mouth and nose. Breathe in slowly. Also apply it to your feet and the back of your neck.[2]

2. Encourages Lymphatic Drainage

Apply 2 to 3 drops to your feet before bedtime or combine 3 to 5 drops with a carrier oil for a calming and relaxing massage and to encourage lymphatic drainage.

3. Helps Digestive System

To support digestion and regulate appetite, rub 3 to 5 drops of bergamot oil onto your stomach. This may stimulate muscle contractions in your intestines and the production of digestive juices.

2. Russo, R., Cassiano, M.G.V., Ciociaro, A., Adornetto, A., Varano, G.P., Chiappini, C., Berliocchi, L., Tassorelli, C., Bagetta, G., Tiziana Corasaniti, M. (2014, November 24). Role of D-Limonene in Autophagy Induced by Bergamot Essential Oil in SH-SY5Y Neuroblastoma Cells. *PLoS One*. Retrieved from http://www.ncbi.nlm.nih.gov/pmc/articles/PMC4242674/

4. Acts as a Natural Deodorant

Add bergamot oil to deodorant or apply it directly to your armpits to help prevent the growth of germs that cause body odor. Combine bergamot oil with lemon, cedarwood or sandalwood oils to make a personalized fragrance.[3]

5. Aids in Reducing Stress

Relieve stress and anxiety by using bergamot oil in a diffuser. It can also be applied topically to help with stress by rubbing 1 to 2 drops onto your temples and wrists.

6. Manages Food Cravings

Diffuse in the classroom, at work or at home in between meals to help control hunger pangs.

7. Supports Immunity

To fight harmful bacteria and stress that can lead to illness, take bergamot oil internally, diffuse it, inhale it directly or add a few drops to a warm-water bath.

3. (2011). Health Benefits of Bergamot Essential Oil. *Organic Facts*. Retrieved from https://www.organicfacts.net/health-benefits/essential-oils/health-benefits-of-bergamot-essential-oil.html

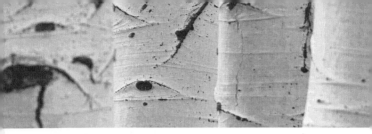

SUPER 7 RX USES
BIRCH

1. Soothes Muscle Pain and Spasms

Birch oil has analgesic properties—it may help relieve muscle and joint pain and aid in alleviating spasms, headaches and toothaches. Apply it topically to the area of concern. For toothaches, apply 1 to 2 drops to the outside of your mouth.

2. Relieves Arthritis Symptoms

Birch essential oil may improve circulation and has detoxifying agents that aid in reducing swelling, rheumatism and arthritis. Apply it topically to the area of concern.[4]

3. Helps Reduce Chronic Inflammation Associated with Gout

Because birch oil helps alleviate inflammation, it may be useful to those suffering from gout. Apply 3 to 4 drops to the affected areas to help ease some of the pain associated with gout.

---

4. Dehelean, C.A., Şoica, C., Ledeţi, I., Aluaş, M., Zupko, I., Găluşcan, A., Cinta-Pinzaru, S., Munteanu, M. (2012, November 19). Study of the betulin enriched birch bark extracts effects on human carcinoma cells and ear inflammation. *Chem Cent J.* Retrieved from http://www.ncbi.nlm.nih.gov/pmc/articles/PMC3527166/

4. May Relieve Pain from Ulcers and Cramps

Due to its anti-spasmodic properties, birch oil assists in relieving pain from ulcers and cramps throughout the body. Apply 2 to 3 drops with a carrier oil to the abdomen, or add 3 to 5 drops to a warm-water bath.

5. Can Improve Mood and Self-Esteem

Birch oil stimulates the nervous, sensory and circulatory systems. It is warming and can provide a sense of peace, confidence and awareness. Diffuse birch oil or apply it topically to your wrists, the back of your neck and the soles of your feet.

6. Encourages Improved Circulation

Birch oil stimulates the circulatory system and can improve circulation. To encourage blood flow, apply to areas of poor circulation.

7. Supports Kidney Detox

Because birch oil is both diuretic and stimulant in nature, it aids in the removal of toxins through increased urination and perspiration. Dilute birch with a carrier oil and massage it into your skin to support kidney detox.

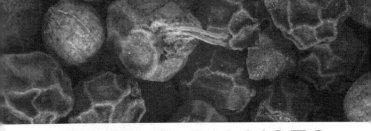

SUPER 7 RX USES
BLACK PEPPER

1. Aids Circulation

To increase circulation and blood flow to the muscles and nerves, add 3 to 5 drops of black pepper oil to a warm compress and apply to your abdomen or area of concern.

2. Improves Digestion

Black pepper may help ease the discomfort of constipation, diarrhea and gas. Take 1 to 2 drops of black pepper oil internally by adding it to a smoothie, soup or savory dish. It can also be applied topically to your abdomen.[5]

3. Helps Soothe Sprains and Tendonitis

Because of its warming, anti-inflammatory and anti-spasmodic properties, black pepper oil works to reduce muscle injuries and tendonitis. Apply topically to the area of concern.

5. McNamara, F.N., Randall, A., Gunthorpe, M.J. (2005, March). Effects of piperine, the pungent component of black pepper, at the human vanilloid receptor (TRPV1). Br J Pharmacol. Retrieved from http://www .ncbi.nlm.nih.gov/pmc/articles/PMC1576058/

4. Aids Respiratory Conditions

Black pepper oil supports the draining and cleansing of your respiratory and lymphatic systems. You can either take it internally or inhale the oil. To relieve congested airways, apply 2 to 3 drops topically to your chest.

5. Helps Reduce Cigarette Cravings

Black pepper oil may help reduce cravings for cigarettes and symptoms of anxiety in smokers deprived from smoking. Inhale or diffuse the oil to help with cravings.

6. Relieves Symptoms of Arthritis and Rheumatism

Due to its warming, anti-inflammatory and circulating properties, black pepper oil helps relieve symptoms of arthritis and rheumatism. Apply topically to the area of concern.

7. Helps to Detoxify the Body

Black pepper oil increases sweating and urination—helping to remove bodily toxins and excess water. This reduces swelling and inflammation and can lower blood pressure. Take internally or apply 2 to 3 drops topically to the soles of your feet.

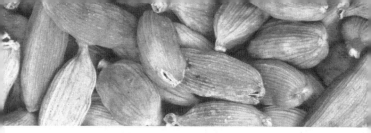

SUPER 7 RX USES
CARDAMOM

1. Helps Ease Digestive Concerns

Cardamom oil calms and promotes digestion, assists in alleviating discomfort from intestinal illnesses and helps reduce symptoms of vomiting, nausea and diarrhea. It may also help with loss of appetite. Take 1 to 3 drops internally, or apply it topically to your abdomen.

2. Diminishes Menstrual and PMS Symptoms

Apply 3 to 4 drops topically to your abdomen to help relieve some of the discomfort associated with menstruation and PMS.

3. Improves Sore Throat

Apply cardamom oil to your chest to soothe a sore throat. The oil's warming properties heat up the body, promote sweating and help clear congestion and coughs that may lead to a sore throat.

4. Serves as a Natural Aphrodisiac

Diffusing cardamom oil or applying 1 to 2 drops topically can have an arousing effect, making it helpful for impotence, erectile dysfunction, loss of libido and frigidity. It stimulates and invigorates the senses while working as a relaxing and warming agent.

5. Lessens Muscle Pain and Cramps

Because of cardamom's anti-spasmodic and anti-inflammatory properties, it helps relieve muscle and joint pain, which could alleviate some of the symptoms of arthritis, menopause and menstruation. Apply it topically to the area of concern.

6. Decreases Mental Fatigue and Brain Fog

Cardamom can clear the mind and ease mental fatigue because of its stimulating and invigorating properties. Apply 1 to 2 drops topically under your nose and the back of your neck.

7. Freshens Breath

Because of cardamom's antiseptic and anti-microbial properties, it can be used as a mouthwash to eliminate bad breath and reduce oral cavities. Add a few drops to water and swish in your mouth.

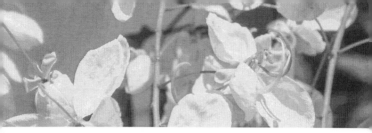

SUPER 7 RX USES
CASSIA

1. Promotes Healthy Blood Sugar Levels

Studies suggest that cassia oil has the ability to naturally improve diabetes by helping to lower blood sugar levels. To support healthy blood sugar levels, take 1 drop of cassia oil internally with tea, coffee, oatmeal or any dish that has a warm and spicy flavor.

2. Boosts Metabolism

Cassia oil can act as a stimulant. Rub 2 to 4 drops of cassia oil onto the soles of your feet or abdomen in order to give your metabolism a boost.

3. Warms Cold Extremities

Rub a few drops of cassia oil on your legs and the soles of your feet or add 5 to 7 drops to a warm-water bath to encourage warmth and stimulate cold extremities.

4. Boosts Libido

Diffuse or put 2 drops of cassia oil on a handkerchief and inhale the scent to give your libido a boost.

5. Encourages Lung Detoxification

Diffuse or put cassia oil in a handkerchief and inhale to promote lung detoxification.

6. Reduces Food Cravings

Combine 1 drop along with a drop of lemon oil in a glass of water and consume to aid digestion and ward off hunger cravings.

7. Acts as a Natural Anti-depressant

To fight harmful bacteria and Cassia contains cinnamaldehyde, a component that has been studied and is known to alleviate stress-induced behaviors and conditions. Diffuse cassia oil or add it to a warm-water bath.[6]

6. Yao, Y., Huang, H.Y., Yang, Y.X., Guo, J.Y. (2015, March 13). Cinnamic aldehyde treatment alleviates chronic unexpected stress-induced depressive-like behaviors via targeting cyclooxygenase-2 in mid-aged rats. *J Ethnopharmacol*. Retrieved from http://www.ncbi.nlm.nih.gov/pubmed/25556926

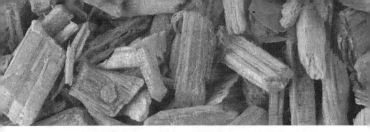

SUPER 7 RX USES
CEDARWOOD

1. **Improves Focus and Eases Symptoms of ADD/ ADHD**

Inhaling cedarwood oil may improve focus and ease symptoms of ADHD. For children with ADHD, an important study by Dr. Terry Friedmann proved that taking three deep inhalations of a blend that included cedarwood oil for 30 days showed significant improvements.

2. **Improves Acne and Eczema**

Cedarwood oil can treat inflammation that leads to irritating skin issues such as eczema. It reduces skin peeling and treats infections with its anti-fungal properties. To improve acne naturally, add 2 to 3 drops of cedarwood oil to lotion or massage it directly into your skin.

3. **Sharpens Focus and Concentration**

Add 2 to 3 drops to skin lotion or soap to enhance your focus. You can also inhale it directly from the bottle or diffuse it.

4. Provides Cough and Sinus Relief

Help remove phlegm from your respiratory tract and lungs by rubbing cedarwood oil onto your chest and throat. Inhaling the oil may also reduce congestion.

5. Repels Insects

Apply cedarwood oil topically to drive away mosquitoes, flies and other insects. It can also be added to water and sprayed on beds and couches. To keep moths away, add 3 drops to cotton balls and leave them around the house.

6. Helps Relieve Tension

Cedarwood oil has a soothing and calming effect on the mind and helps ease tight muscles. Add the oil to a diffuser, inhale it directly from the bottle or apply it topically.

7. Fights Fungal Infections

Applying cedarwood oil topically or diffusing it aids in protecting the body from fungal pathogens and internal and external infections.

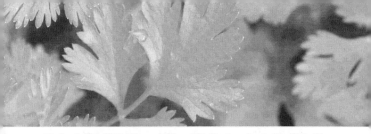

SUPER 7 RX USES
CILANTRO

1. **Supports Heavy Metal Detox**

Cilantro essential oil has been shown to bind toxic metals together—loosening them from tissue and facilitating their elimination from the body. Ingest 1 to 2 drops at a time or diffuse the oil.

2. **Supports Healthy Liver Function**

To support healthy liver function, take 1 to 2 drops of cilantro internally in food or liquid, apply it topically to your abdomen or diffuse it.

3. **Helps Settle the Stomach**

Cilantro oil can help settle nausea, prevent gas and bloating, relieve indigestion and heartburn and ease stomach cramps. It may also protect the body against food poisoning because of its anti-microbial properties. Apply 3 to 5 drops topically to your stomach.

4. Supports Anti-Aging

Cilantro has antioxidant properties that protect the body against damage caused by free radicals. Diffuse cilantro oil around your home to support the reduction of oxidative stress.

5. Encourages Proper Blood Sugar Levels

Cilantro helps to balance blood sugar levels. As needed, ingest 1 to 3 drops of cilantro oil as a natural support for diabetes.

6. Supports Cardiovascular Disease Protection

Cilantro oil has polyphenolic content and natural cardio-protective nutrients responsible for preventing oxidative damage that is directly associated with cardiac damage. Ingest 1 drop of cilantro oil for protection.

7. May Prevent Urinary Tract Infections

Cilantro oil's anti-bacterial compounds help to keep the urinary tract healthy and free from germs that cause UTIs. Take internally or apply it to your abdomen.

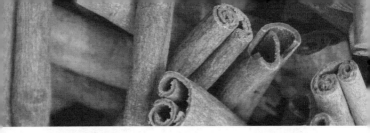

SUPER 7 RX USES
CINNAMON BARK

1. Boosts Heart Health

Because of its circulation-boosting abilities, cinnamon oil can support the cleansing of arteries. Apply 2 to 3 drops of cinnamon oil mixed with ½ teaspoon of coconut oil to your chest to promote warmth and increased blood flow.

2. Supports Healthy Blood Sugar and Insulin Release

Cinnamon oil may help keep blood sugar stable and prevent chronic fatigue, moodiness, sugar cravings and overeating. Inhale cinnamon essential oil, diffuse it or apply it to your chest and wrists.

3. May Help with High Cholesterol

One study revealed that a key constituent in cinnamon bark oil, cinnamate, lowers the activity of an enzyme that makes cholesterol in the body called HMG CoA reductase—the same enzyme targeted by statins. Take 1 to 2 drops of cinnamon essential oil internally to fight high cholesterol.

4. Helps Fight Infections

Diffusing cinnamon bark essentialoil has shown an inhibitory effect against respiratory tract pathogens, including some penicillin-resistant strains. Diffuse it daily for protection against infection or to relieve a present infection.

5. Promotes Weight Loss

Because cinnamon oil can balance blood sugar levels and improve the taste of foods without added sugar, it's effective for curbing a sweet tooth. Add 1 to 2 drops to fruit, oats, baked goods or smoothies to help slow the rate at which glucose is released into the blood.

6. Fights Parasites

Studies have found that cinnamon oil inhibits the growth of certain harmful parasites. Ingest the oil to fight harmful parasites and impede parasite growth.

7. Soothes Sore Throat

Cinnamon oil can help prevent mucus buildup and clear nasal passages. Drink hot lemon water, honey and 1 drop of cinnamon oil in the morning to soothe a sore throat (plus curb cravings and support immune function).

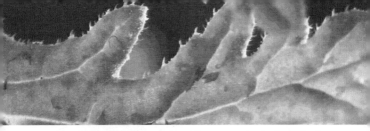

SUPER 7 RX USES
CITRONELLA

1. Repels Insects

Citronella effectively repels mosquitoes, body lice, head lice and flies. Combine 3 to 5 drops of citronella oil with coconut oil and spread it on your body like a lotion, or add the oil to a spray bottle filled with water and spray it on your clothes, skin and furniture.

2. Helps Reduce Pain and Swelling

Due to its antioxidant properties and ability to increase blood flow, citronella is used as a natural support for arthritis. Massage 3 to 5 drops onto swollen joints, tissue and muscles, or soak in a warm bath with 5 drops of citronella oil.

3. Relaxes the Body and Mind

Citronella oil has relaxing properties that can help reduce stress and aid sleep. Diffuse citronella or massage citronella oil into your skin, specifically on the back of your neck.

4. Detoxifies the Body/Kidneys

Citronella oil can increase sweating and urination, which draws toxins out of the body. Combine 2 drops with a teaspoon of raw honey, 2 drops of lemon oil and hot water. Mix well and drink. This combination may improve the elimination of excess fats, sodium, uric acid and toxins.

5. Cleans and Deodorizes the Home

Deodorize the home and help kill bacteria and fungi with citronella oil. Add to a spray bottle filled with water and use the mixture on kitchen and household appliances. Adding citronella oil to the dishwasher, refrigerator and laundry machine is also effective.

6. Calms Pets

Combine 3 drops of citronella oil with coconut oil, and then massage the mixture into small areas on your pet's skin. Citronella oil can also be added to a clean cotton swab and applied topically to calm a nervous pet.

7. Supports Hair Health

Citronella oil can eliminate excess oil and greasiness from the hair while also adding shine and fighting dandruff. Add 5 to 7 drops to a bottle of shampoo or conditioner or combine with 1 teaspoon of coconut oil and massage the mixture into your hair and scalp.

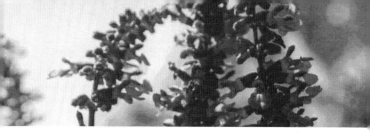

SUPER 7 RX USES
CLARY SAGE

1. **Supports Hormonal Balance**

Clary sage oil contains natural phytoestrogens, which give it the ability to produce estrogenic effects. The oil can help regulate estrogen levels and support the long-term health of the uterus. To help balance hormones, apply 3 drops regularly to your abdomen, 2 drops to your neck or diffuse the oil.

2. Helps with Menstrual Discomfort

Clary sage oil has the power to alleviate some of the symptoms of PMS. It is also anti-spasmodic, meaning it can treat spasms and muscle cramps. To relieve menstrual discomfort, take it internally or apply it topically to your abdomen.

3. Promotes Restfulness

Clary sage oil is a natural sedative. To help relieve insomnia and feelings of anxiety, diffuse it at your bedside or rub 1 to 2 drops onto your neck and the soles of your feet.

4. Supports Healthy Circulation

By opening up the blood vessels and allowing for increased blood circulation, clary sage oil may be beneficial to the heart. It also naturally lowers blood pressure by relaxing the brain and arteries. Rub the oil onto your limbs and chest.

5. May Help Lower Cholesterol

The anti-inflammatory and antioxidant properties of clary sage oil may help to lower cholesterol naturally. Diffuse it or add 5 drops to a warm-water bath.

6. Contains Compounds Beneficial for Fighting Leukemia

A chemical compound found in clary sage oil, called sclareol, is able to kill leukemia cell lines through apoptosis. An insufficient amount of apoptosis results in uncontrolled abnormal cell proliferation, i.e. cancer. Take clary sage oil internally to promote apoptosis.

7. Boosts Skin Health

An important ester in clary sage oil, called linalyl acetate, has been shown to reduce skin inflammation and work as a natural remedy for rashes. Combine clary sage oil with jojoba oil and apply it to your skin.

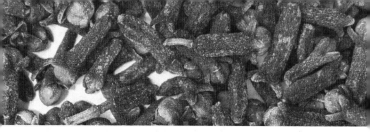

SUPER 7 RX USES
CLOVE

1. Helps Fight Candida

Clove is an anti-fungal agent, and studies show that it is equally as effective as nystatin, a drug commonly prescribed to manage yeast infections of the mouth (thrush). Place 1 drop of clove oil in a capsule or mix it into your food or beverage and consume daily for up to two weeks to fight candida.

2. Promotes Oral Health

Clove is widely accepted as a reliable solution for dry sockets and to relieve the pain and discomfort associated with various dental disorders. It also slows tooth decalcification, or dental erosion. Dilute 1 to 2 drops with equal parts coconut oil and apply to the affected area.

3. Battles Parasites

Take clove oil internally for up to two weeks, either mixed with a carrier oil or in capsules, to rid the body of unwanted parasites.

4. Helps Prevent Oxidative Stress

Research has shown that clove contains an astounding amount of antioxidants that slow aging. To prevent damage caused by free radicals, diffuse it or dilute it with a carrier oil and apply it topically to your neck and chest.

5. May Improve Acne

Clove oil is a powerful anti-bacterial agent that can help eliminate acne and skin infections. Mix 3 drops of clove oil with 2 teaspoons of raw honey. Apply the mixture to your face, let it sit for a few minutes and then rinse off and pat dry.

6. Fights Cold and Flu Viruses

The anti-viral properties in clove essential oil help boost the immune system. Clove oil has the power to purify blood, thereby increasing the resistance to diseases and infections. To boost the immune system, diffuse clove oil or apply it topically with carrier oil.

7. Supports Healthy Blood Pressure Levels

To ease feelings of stress and uneasiness and to lower elevated blood pressure associated with stress, diffuse clove oil at home or dilute it with coconut oil and apply to your wrists.

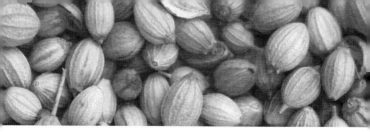

SUPER 7 RX USES
CORIANDER

1. **Supports Healthy Blood Sugar Levels**

Coriander contains compounds that lead to a wide array of pharmacological activities, including its ability to potentially assist with lowering cholesterol, blood pressure and blood sugar levels. To support healthy blood sugar, take 1 drop internally as needed.

2. **Eases Gas, Nausea and Bloating**

Coriander oil's digestive and anti-spasmodic properties aid in relieving gas and nausea; it helps to relax the digestive system and may ease irritability that can lead to nausea. Apply 2 to 3 drops topically to your abdomen, or take 1 drop internally.

3. **Helps with Rashes and Skin Irritation**

Coriander oil is considered an effective Ayurvedic remedy for rashes and itchy skin, due to its anti-irritant, soothing, anti-inflammatory and antiseptic properties. Apply 2 to 3 drops topically to the area of concern.

4. Eases Anxiety

Coriander oil is a mild stimulant, and it is capable of relaxing the mind—reducing feelings of stress and nervousness. Diffuse or apply a blend of coriander, lavender and Roman chamomile topically to the soles of your feet and the back of your neck.

5. Helps Alleviate Muscle and Joint Pain

Because of its anti-inflammatory and anti-spasmodic properties, coriander oil may reduce pain associated with arthritis, rheumatism, stiffness and gout. For soothing relief, apply it topically to the area of concern.

6. May Help with Adrenal Fatigue

To naturally support your adrenals and promote proper function, apply coriander to the back of your neck or the soles of your feet.

7. Stimulates Appetite

To boost appetite and help battle anorexia, take 1 drop of coriander oil internally or apply 2 to 3 drops to your palms, cup your nose and inhale deeply for 5 minutes.

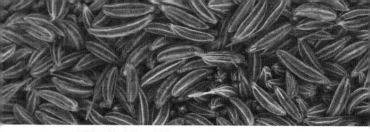

SUPER 7 RX USES
CUMIN

1. Aids Digestion

Cumin oil promotes the discharge of bile and gastric juices when taken in small doses, which can help the digestive system. It can also prevent the formation of gas. Take 1 drop of cumin oil by adding it to food to help relieve digestive issues.

2. Assists in Detoxifying the Body

Cumin oil is a diuretic and may stimulate urination, which helps the body to flush out excess water, salt and toxins. Take 1 drop of cumin oil internally to detoxify your body.

3. May Prevent Infections

Cumin oil has antiseptic and anti-bacterial properties, so it may help to prevent infections and bacterial overgrowth. It can be used on both internal and external wounds and cuts. Dilute 2 to 3 drops and apply to the infection, or take 1 drop internally for infections.

4. Relieves Cramps and Spasms

Because of its anti-spasmodic properties, cumin oil can help to relieve cramps and spasms due to menstruation and issues such as digestive spasms and restless legs syndrome. Apply cumin oil topically to the area of concern.

5. Tones Skin, Muscles and Organs

Cumin works as a tonic, so it has the ability to tone various systems in the body, including the nervous, digestive, circulatory and excretory systems. Massage 2 to 4 drops of cumin oil and 1 teaspoon of coconut oil onto the soles of your feet to stimulate bodily organs.

6. Regulates Menstruation Cycle

Cumin oil works as an emmenagogue—meaning it helps to maintain a regular menstrual cycle by opening obstructed menses. Apply it topically over your uterus, inhale from the bottle deeply 10 times or take it internally.

7. Supports Nerve Tissue

Cumin oil is good for nerves and supports nervous disorders such as convulsions, anxiety and stress. Add 1 drop to your favorite dish for added flavor and benefit, or diffuse it.

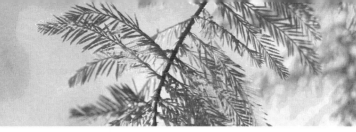

SUPER 7 RX USES
CYPRESS

1. Reduces the Appearance of Varicose Veins and Cellulite

Cypress essential oil stimulates blood flow and relieves fluid retention—alleviating the causes of varicose veins and cellulite. Apply 2 to 4 drops along with a carrier oil to the areas of concern.

2. Helps Diminish Hemorrhoids

Cypress essential oil is known as an effective oil for reducing and preventing hemorrhoids. Apply 3 to 4 drops with a cotton ball.

3. Eases Restless Leg Syndrome

When used topically, cypress oil may help reduce the discomfort associated with restless leg syndrome and could help increase blood circulation. Apply it topically to the area of concern.

4. Lessens Swelling from Sprains and Strains

Because of cypress oil's anti-spasmodic qualities, it helps inhibit problems associated with spasms, such as cramps and muscle strains. Apply it topically to areas of concern.

5. Supports a Healthy Prostate

Cypress oil may help reduce the size of an enlarged prostate. The applications most commonly used for prostate conditions are bath, massage blend or suppository. For suppository use, contact a clinically trained and registered aromatherapist.

6. Helps with Edema and Fluid Retention

Cypress oil is a diuretic, so it helps the body flush out internal toxins. It also increases sweat and perspiration, which allows the body to quickly remove toxins, excess salt and water. Apply it topically to your wrists, the back of your neck, abdomen and the soles of your feet.

7. Calms Respiratory Conditions

Cypress oil calms the respiratory system and works as an anti-spasmodic agent—helping to relieve respiratory conditions such as asthma and bronchitis. To remedy respiratory conditions, add 5 drops to a warm-water bath, or dilute it and apply the mixture to your chest to work as a vapor rub.

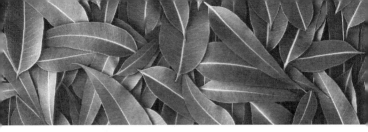

SUPER 7 RX USES
EUCALYPTUS

1. Helps Ease Symptoms of Bronchitis & Pneumonia

Eucalyptus can ease symptoms of respiratory conditions by dilating the blood vessels and allowing more oxygen into the lungs. Mix 3 to 5 drops with equal parts of peppermint and coconut oil to make a homemade vapor rub; rub the mixture onto your chest.

2. Reduces Earaches

Eucalyptus can be an effective treatment for earaches. Add several drops of eucalyptus oil to a pan of boiling water, remove the pan from the heat, place a towel over your head and inhale the steam. Also try gently massaging the oil into the skin around your ear.

3. Helps Improve Asthma and Allergies

Studies show that eucalyptus oil is effective at treating sinusitis and that patients sometimes experience faster improvement when using the oil for allergies, breathing and sinus issues. Gargle with 1 to 2 drops of eucalyptus oil or apply it topically to your chest.

4. Promotes Energy and Focus

To feel energized, alert and focused, diffuse eucalyptus throughout your home or at work, or rub a few drops on your temples or neck.

5. Provides Relief from Shingles

Eucalyptus oil may help with the pain associated with shingles. Apply eucalyptus to your skin for instant relief from itching and pain.

6. Serves as a Cleaning Aid

Because of its anti-microbial properties, eucalyptus oil can help disinfect the home. Put 10 to 15 drops into home-care products such as laundry detergent and toilet cleaner. It can also be added to vacuums or a diffuser to inhibit the growth of mold and bacteria in the home.

7. Aids in Wound Care

Because of its anti-microbial and antiseptic properties, eucalyptus oil effectively treats wounds, burns, cuts, insect stings, abrasions, sores and scrapes. It also fights infections and may speed healing. Apply eucalyptus oil to the affected area twice daily.

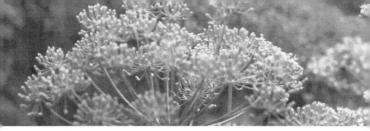

SUPER 7 RX USES
FENNEL

1. Aids Digestion

Fennel essential oil aids digestion by stimulating the secretion of digestive juices. It can also help balance the pH level within the stomach, thereby reducing acid reflux after meals. Fennel oil may also be used to treat intestinal parasites and sluggish bowels. Take 1 to 2 drops internally by adding the oil to water or tea, or take it in a capsule.

2. Improves Colic

Fennel seed oil has been shown to reduce colic pain and increase motility in the small intestine. The safest way to reduce colic pain is for a breastfeeding mother to drink fennel tea. Alternatively, 1 diluted drop can be applied topically to the baby's abdomen.

3. Prevents Edema and Fluid Retention

Fennel essential oil is a natural diuretic and can be used to prevent the retention of fluid within the body. Combine 1 to 2 drops of fennel oil with equal parts of grapefruit oil and rub the mixture onto the affected area.

4. Eases PMS and Menstrual Symptoms

Fennel essential oil is anti-spasmodic and may reduce uterine contraction frequency and intensity. Take 1 to 2 drops by adding it to tea or water. Fennel oil may also be applied topically to your abdomen to help tone female organs and support healthy menstruation.

5. Relieves Symptoms of Menopause

Research suggests fennel oil has potential in preventing bone loss in women with postmenopausal osteoporosis. It also helps to maintain emotional balance as well as promote healthy hormone levels. Take it internally, or apply it topically to your abdomen.[7]

6. Stimulates the Flow of Breast Milk

Fennel oil helps promote a healthy balance of hormones and may support the flow of breast milk in women with low milk supply. Take it internally or drink fennel tea.

7. Lessens Gas and Bloating

Taking fennel essential oil internally promotes healthy digestion and may help to relieve hunger pains.

7. Mahmoudi, Z., Soleimani, M., Saidi, A., Khamisipour, G., Azizsoltani, A. (2013). Effects of Foeniculum vulgare ethanol extract on osteogenesis in human mecenchymal stem cells. *Avicenna J Phytomed*. Retrieved from http://www.ncbi.nlm.nih.gov/pmc/articles/PMC4075705/

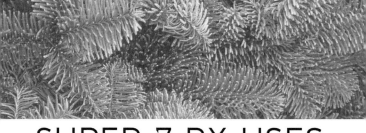

SUPER 7 RX USES
FIR NEEDLE

1. Helps with Respiratory Issues

Fir needle oil can be very helpful for respiratory issues that accompany the common cold and flu. Add 5 drops of fir needle oil to your diffuser and breathe in some natural relief.

2. Aids in Healing Broken Bones

Fir needle oil can assist in bone repair. Dilute it with a carrier oil (such as coconut oil) and apply it to the problematic area three times per day.

3. Helps with Ligament Tears

Fir needle oil may help speed the healing of ligament tears. Apply it topically to the affected area to help speed recovery.

4. Displays Anti-tumor Properties

Fir needle essential oil has been found to be an efficient anti-cancer agent, which may make it an effective supplement to take for cancerous tumors. Take 1 to 2 drops internally, or massage the oil onto the affected area to support beneficial tumor and anti-cancer response.

5. Provides Pain Relief

Fir needle essential oil makes an excellent analgesic. To help relax muscles and soothe body aches—important for muscle recovery—apply it topically to aching muscles and body aches.

6. Cleans and Sanitizes the House

Fir needle makes an excellent addition to homemade cleaning solutions. The next time you're creating an all-purpose cleaner, add a few drops of fir needle oil for a natural yet powerful disinfecting boost.

7. May Help Prevent Osteoporosis

When applied topically, essential oils such as fir, cypress and helichrysum may help to increase bone density. Dilute it with a carrier oil and apply to the area of concern.

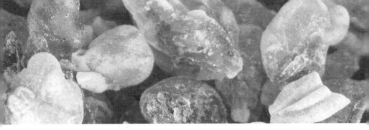

SUPER 7 RX USES
FRANKINCENSE

1. Serves as a Powerful Addition to Cancer-Fighting Protocols

Frankincense essential oil has been shown to help fight specific types of cancer cells. Take 2 to 3 drops internally, use as a suppository (under the supervision of a health practitioner) or massage the oil onto the affected area to support healthy immune system response.

2. May Relieve Joint Inflammation and Pain

To improve circulation and help relieve symptoms of joint or muscle pain related to conditions such as arthritis, digestive disorders and asthma, massage frankincense oil onto the painful area or diffuse.

3. Boosts the Immune System

Studies have demonstrated that frankincense has immune-enhancing abilities. It can be used to prevent germs from forming on the skin, in the mouth or in the home. Diffuse it, take it internally or rub onto your temples, wrists and the soles of your feet.

4. Promotes Relaxation During Meditation and Prayer

Frankincense oil may help induce a feeling of peace and relaxation, making it ideal for prayer time and meditation. Diffuse it during meditation and anoint your family with this ancient, powerful oil.

5. Relieves Cold and Flu Symptoms

Frankincense oil can help eliminate phlegm in the lungs and acts as an anti-inflammatory agent in the nasal passages. To treat respiratory conditions, add 5 drops of frankincense oil to a diffuser and breathe in deeply for 5 minutes, or rub 2 to 3 drops onto your chest.

6. Reduces the Appearance of Stretch Marks and Wrinkles

Frankincense oil can help minimize stretch marks, scars and wrinkles. Mix 2 to 3 drops of the oil with equal parts of coconut or jojoba oil and apply to the affected areas.

7. Helps Those with Brain Injury and Alzheimer's

Because it improves cognitive health and responses, frankincense oil may be used on people with Alzheimer's disease, dementia and brain injury. Take it internally, diffuse it, or apply it topically to the back of your neck and under your nose.

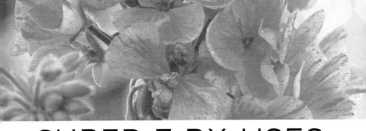

SUPER 7 RX USES
GERANIUM

1. **Promotes Radiant, Youthful Skin**

Because geranium oil is an astringent, it induces contractions, which improves skin tone. It has the power to minimize the appearance of wrinkles and can help slow down the effects of aging. Add 2 drops to facial lotion or equal parts of coconut oil and apply it twice daily.

2. **Helps Balance Hormones**

Geranium can regulate hormone levels and help ease the symptoms of PMS and menstruation. Apply 1 to 2 drops topically to your abdomen along with clary sage oil, orange oil and a carrier oil just prior to the onset of your menstrual cycle.

3. **Aids in Cleaning the Kidneys**

Geranium oil is a natural diuretic, meaning it may increase urination, thereby helping to eliminate toxins from the body. Take it internally, or apply it topically to your abdomen.

4. Promotes Healthy Muscle Toning

Geranium oil helps to tighten and contract muscles. As a result, it can help prevent muscles and skin from sagging, and its use may result in a more toned abdomen. Create a massage oil by mixing 5 drops of geranium oil with 1 tablespoon of jojoba oil.

5. Reduces the Appearance of Eczema and Psoriasis

Geranium oil has anti-inflammatory and moisturizing properties that can aid in the repair of red, dry, flaking skin. Mix geranium oil with shea butter and apply it to any damaged skin.

6. Induces Blood Clotting

Geranium oil causes the contraction of blood vessels and helps to stop blood flow; it also speeds up the formation of blood clots. This aids in healing wounds or incisions, and it keeps toxins from entering the body.

7. May Help Prevent Alzheimer's and Dementia

Geranium oil works with the natural chemistry of the brain to help prevent conditions that can lead to memory loss. Rub the oil onto your temples, wrists and the back of your neck.

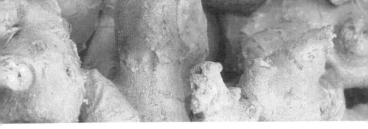

SUPER 7 RX USES
GINGER

1. Helps Ease Nausea and Morning Sickness

Ginger essential oil is effective as a natural remedy for nausea and vomiting. To relieve nausea and vomiting, diffuse 2 to 3 drops or apply 1 to 2 drops topically onto your stomach.

2. Promotes Digestion

Ginger essential oil is one of the best natural remedies for colic, indigestion, diarrhea, spasms and stomachaches. Rub a few drops of ginger oil with a carrier oil on your abdomen, inhale it directly or add 1 drop to your food or beverage.

3. Aids in Healing Infections

Ginger oil is an antiseptic, fighting a broad spectrum of infections. This includes intestinal infections, bacterial dysentery and food poisoning. For external infections, apply 2 to 3 drops topically to the affected area. For internal infections, consume it by adding it to tea, water or food. Add one drop at a time, tasting between drops for tolerance.

4. Eases Colds and Sore Throats

Ginger essential oil helps remove mucus from the throat and lungs. It also naturally aids in relieving coughs, asthma and bronchitis and helps with loss of breath. Add 1 drop of ginger essential oil to a cup of green tea twice daily. It can also be applied topically to your chest.

5. Reduces Inflammation and Joint Pain

A component of ginger essential oil, called zingibain, is responsible for the oil's anti-inflammatory properties. This component provides pain relief and treats muscle aches, arthritis, headaches and migraines. To reduce inflammation, take 1 to 3 drops of ginger oil internally once a day, or apply 2 drops topically to the affected area.

6. Helps Relieve Anxiety

Ginger oil may be able to relieve feelings of anxiety, depression and exhaustion. The warming quality of ginger oil acts as a sleep aid and stimulates feelings of courage and ease. Use the oil aromatically by diffusing 3 to 5 drops, or add 5 drops to a warm-water bath.

7. May Alleviate Pain from Sprains and Strains

Research suggests that consuming ginger essential oil daily is more effective in treating muscle and joint pain than some prescription painkillers. Apply to the affected area or add to warm bath water.

SUPER 7 RX USES
GRAPEFRUIT

1. May Boost Weight Loss

Grapefruit oil can support metabolism and may reduce appetite. Mix grapefruit oil with patchouli oil and diffuse it. To boost your metabolism, add 2 drops to water, a smoothie or sparkling beverage. Also massage the oil onto your chest and wrists when a craving strikes.

2. Curbs Food Cravings

Grapefruit is known to lower sugar cravings and help kick sugar addiction when inhaled. Add several drops to a cotton ball along with a touch of coconut oil; then rub it onto your wrists, neck or chest, or inhale it directly to stave off cravings.

3. Promotes Lymphatic Drainage

Grapefruit oil is an excellent diuretic and lymphatic stimulant, making it effective for shedding excess water weight; it can also help eliminate toxins and excess salt. Take 1 to 2 drops internally, or apply it topically over your kidneys.

4. Helps with Gallbladder Function and Fat Digestion

By increasing blood to the digestive organs, grapefruit oil helps with detoxification. It has a positive effect on digestion, can help reduce fluid retention and fights microbes within the intestines, gut and other digestive organs. Make a homemade massage lotion with grapefruit and coconut or jojoba oil, and then rub the mixture onto your abdomen.

5. Fights Candida

Grapefruit essential oil has anti-fungal abilities and is able to reduce yeast and bacteria. Research shows that grapefruit is also effective at fighting urinary tract infections. Diffuse 5 drops, or take 1 to 2 drops internally.

6. Freshens the Air

To get rid of unpleasant odors, diffuse grapefruit oil along with other citrus scents such as lemon oil and orange oil. Additionally, use grapefruit oil on wooden surfaces, countertops, floors or household appliances to help kill bacteria and mask odor.

7. Helps Reduce the Appearance of Cellulite

Grapefruit essential oil helps to reduce inflammation and increase blood flow, which may lessen the appearance of cellulite. Rub a mixture of grapefruit oil and coconut oil onto areas of concern daily.

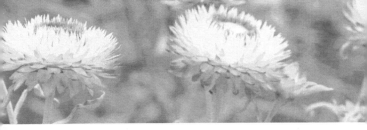

SUPER 7 RX USES
HELICHRYSUM

1. May Ease Nerve Pain

Helichrysum, especially when combined with frankincense oil, may support the neurological system and can alleviate some of the symptoms of multiple sclerosis. Apply 2 drops of each oil to your temples, wrists and the soles of your feet every day for three weeks. Take one week off and repeat the cycle.

2. Diminishes Bruising and Bleeding

Helichrysum's anti-inflammatory and anti-spasmodic properties help to reduce pain, bruising and swelling. Apply 2 to 3 drops topically to the back of your neck or any area of pain; repeat several times daily.

3. Reduces the Appearance of Wrinkles

Helichrysum hydrates the skin and can decrease signs of aging and block UV damage that can lead to skin cancer. Use helichrysum topically by combining 2 to 3 drops with a carrier oil, and apply it where you are most prone to wrinkles.

4. Acts as a Natural Digestive Aid and Diuretic

Helichrysum helps stimulate the secretion of gastric juices to break down food and prevent indigestion. It also reduces bloating. Rub onto your abdomen or take internally.

5. Detoxifies Liver and Kidney

Known to be an anti-spasmodic agent, blood purifier and anti-inflammatory, helichrysum has been used as a liver and kidney stimulant and detoxifier for centuries. Take internally to promote healthy liver and pancreas function and heavy metal chelation.

6. May Stop Cancer Cell Growth

Helichrysum contains flavonoid antioxidant compounds that inhibit oxidative stress and cancer growth in lab experiments. It may protect cells against radiation-induced DNA damage, cell mutation and death, and cancerous tumor growth. Take it internally by adding the oil to a glass of water or cup of tea.

7. Boosts the Immune System

Because of its gut-healing and anti-inflammatory properties, helichrysum may boost immunity. It inhibits the growth of harmful bacteria, fungi and viruses. Diffuse it or take it internally to promote gut health and immunity.

SUPER 7 RX USES
HOLY BASIL

1. Supports Thyroid Function

Holy basil acts as an adaptogen (helps the body adapt to stress and exerts a normalizing effect upon bodily processes) to modulate the stress response and fight adrenal fatigue. To support proper thyroid function, take 1 to 2 drops internally with a carrier oil or in a glass of water.

2. May Lessen Anxiety

As stated above, holy basil has been traditionally used to support people through times of stress, working as an adaptogen and anxiolytic (decreasing anxiety). Take it internally or rub on your temples to help decrease stress and elevate your mood.

3. Supports the Nervous System

Holy basil has been shown to improve memory and cognition, anxiety and depression, insomnia, migraines and headaches. Apply it topically to your wrists, temples or the soles of your feet to benefit from its many therapeutic properties.

4. Helps Reduce Inflammation

Holy basil possesses anti-inflammatory and immune-boosting properties that can protect the body against fever, pain, stress and inflammation. Make holy basil tea by adding 2 to 3 drops to hot tea, or apply it topically to areas of pain and discomfort.

5. Supports Healthy Blood Glucose Levels

Holy basil is known for its ability to affect blood glucose levels; in fact, many people use it to manage or even help reverse diabetes. Drink holy basil tea once daily to positively influence blood sugar levels and support diabetes management.

6. Can Regulate Cortisol Levels

Holy basil is able to regulate cortisol levels in the body, which are the stress hormones that can hinder learning, memory, immune function, bone density, weight loss and cardiovascular function. Drink holy basil tea or apply it topically.

7. Treats Respiratory Conditions

Components of holy basil leaves provide relief from congestion and other symptoms of respiratory disorders. To treat respiratory conditions, add 2 to 3 drops of holy basil oil to hot water, or apply it topically to the back of your neck, chest and the soles of your feet.

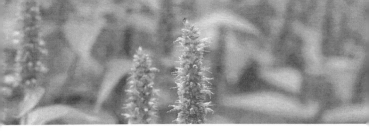

SUPER 7 RX USES
HYSSOP

1. **Helps Relieve Respiratory Conditions**

Hyssop relieves spasms in the respiratory system and soothes coughs. It's also an expectorant, loosening phlegm that has been deposited in the respiratory tract. Hyssop may also reduce lung inflammation. Add 2 to 3 drops to tea, or apply it to your throat and chest.

2. **May Prevent Infections**

Because of its antiseptic properties, hyssop helps prevent infections from developing in wounds and cuts. Hyssop also aids in the healing process of deep cuts, scars, insect bites and acne. Apply it topically to the area of concern.

3. **Fights Parasites**

Hyssop is a vermifuge, which means it has the ability to fight parasites such as tapeworms, hookworms and flukes. Take hyssop oil internally to help rid the body of internal parasites.

4. Encourages Healthy Circulation

By increasing circulation, hyssop can work as a natural treatment for gout, rheumatism, arthritis and swelling. The heart rate lowers when blood circulates properly, thereby relaxing the muscles and regulating blood pressure levels. Consume hyssop oil in tea or hot water to improve circulation.

5. Reduces Muscle Pain and Spasms

Hyssop oil has muscle-relaxing activity, and it may inhibit contractions and spasms that can lead to cramps. Apply 3 to 5 drops topically to the area of concern, or add 5 to 10 drops to a warm-water bath with Epsom salts.

6. Supports a Healthy Immune System

By improving circulation, aiding digestion and helping to prevent infection, hyssop oil supports a healthy immune system. Consume hyssop oil in tea or hot water to boost the immune system.

7. Promotes Skin Health

Hyssop promotes cellular regeneration and the growth of new skin, thereby minimizing the look of scars, stretch marks and wounds. It also helps fight bacteria on the skin. Dilute 2 to 3 drops with a carrier oil and apply it topically to the area of concern.

SUPER 7 RX USES
JASMINE

1. Acts as an Aphrodisiac

Jasmine oil causes increases of the physical signs of arousal, such as breathing rate, body temperature, blood oxygen saturation and systolic and diastolic blood pressure. Diffuse 5 drops of jasmine oil, or apply it topically to the soles of your feet as well as your wrists.

2. Helps Fight Depression and Anxiety

Jasmine oil can improve mood and boost energy levels because of its regenerating and stimulating properties. The oil also has the power to boost concentration and brain activity. Diffuse it, or apply 1 or 3 drops topically to your temples, wrists, the back of your neck or the soles of your feet. Jasmine oil can also be added to a warm bath.

3. Fights Wrinkles and Aging Skin

Jasmine oil displays both antibiotic and anti-viral properties, giving it the ability to help calm skin irritation and inflammation and promote youthful, radiant skin. Mix 1 to 3 drops of jasmine oil into a lip balm, face wash or lotion to fight wrinkles.

4. Acts as a Sleep Aid

Jasmine oil exhibits a calming effect and can act as a natural sedative and help with sleep. Combine jasmine oil with other soothing oils, such as lavender and frankincense, and diffuse it or apply it topically.

5. Eases Feelings of Being Overwhelmed

Jasmine can help ease postpartum symptoms, including anxiety, depression, muscle pain and low energy. It also helps balance hormones naturally and has been used traditionally to increase the production of breast milk. Diffuse jasmine oil or apply it topically.

6. Promotes Hormone Balance

Using jasmine oil may help reduce hot flashes. Diffuse jasmine oil or apply it topically to the back of your neck or the soles of your feet to reduce PMS symptoms, including headaches, stomach cramps, acne and restlessness.

7. Serves as a Mood-Lifting Perfume

Jasmine oil has a warm, flowery smell, similar to many women's perfumes. Apply 1 to 2 drops topically to your wrists, mixed with a carrier oil to tone down the smell. Jasmine oil blends well with vanilla, lavender and orange when making a homemade perfume.

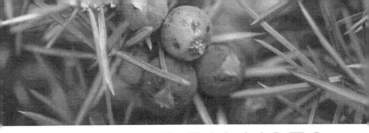

SUPER 7 RX USES
JUNIPER BERRY

1. Soothes and Protects Skin

Juniper berry oil supports healthy skin, helps reduce
the appearance of stretch marks and may treat skin
conditions caused by hormone imbalances. Add 1 to 2
drops to face or body wash, or dilute 2 to 3 drops with a
carrier oil and apply it to the areas of concern.

2. Assists in Cleansing the Liver

Juniper can help stimulate digestive enzymes and make
it easier to break down and absorb protein, fats and
nutrients from foods. For a natural digestive aid or liver
cleanse, add a few drops to a smoothie or glass of water.

3. Boosts Kidney and Urinary Health

Juniper berry oil helps speed up urination and
elimination—drawing out toxins, waste and irritants from
the digestive tract. Apply 1 to 3 drops to your abdomen or
take it internally.

4. Helps Reduce Bloating and Gas

Juniper berries serve as a natural diuretic, which helps the body flush out excess fluids from the bladder and urethra. This process helps reduce bloating and gas. Apply 1 to 3 drops to your abdomen or take it internally.

5. Serves as a Household Cleaner

As a natural antiseptic that can keep certain bacterial strains from spreading within the home, use juniper berry oil on kitchen and bathroom surfaces or appliances. Add 5 drops to the washing machine as a natural alternative to harsh anti-bacterial commercial detergents.

6. Acts as a Sleep Aid

Juniper berry essential oil may relieve muscle tension and prevent restlessness, helping you fall asleep. Diffuse 5 drops before bed, or apply 1 to 3 drops to your neck, chest and the soles of your feet.

7. Soothes Sore Muscles

Juniper berry oil can reduce pain and inflammation, as well as help alleviate pain from injuries and strenuous physical activity. Massage it into the area of concern. It can also be added to bath water, along with lavender oil and Epsom salts.

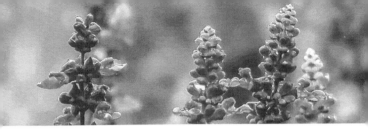

SUPER 7 RX USES
LAVENDER

1. **Promotes Sleep**

To help get a good night's rest, diffuse 5 drops of lavender oil beside your bed, or apply 2 to 3 drops to the back of your neck, as well as your chest and temples.

2. **Soothes Burns, Sunburns and Cuts**

Lavender has been shown to be highly soothing to skin cuts and irritations. Mix lavender oil with coconut oil and apply it to the areas of concern twice daily.

3. **Helps Relieve Anxiety and Stress**

Lavender oil is known to bring on feelings of peace and relaxation. Diffuse lavender oil, add it to a warm-water bath or apply it to your temples, wrists and the soles of your feet.

4. **Combats High Blood Pressure**

Diffuse lavender oil beside you during your workday to help soothe stressed behaviors and promote healthy blood pressure.

5. Stimulates Healthy Blood Sugar Balance

Lavender oil shows promise in protecting the body from increases in blood glucose. Apply it to the back of your neck and your chest, diffuse it or add 1 drop to a glass of water or cup of tea.

6. Helps Relieve Headaches and Migraines

For relief from headache pain, inhale lavender oil for 15 minutes. You can also mix 2 drops of lavender oil with 2 drops of peppermint oil and apply it to the back of your neck and your temples for a tension and pain relief aid.

7. Encourages Healthy Skin

Lavender oil can be applied directly on the skin or mixed with coconut oil for those with sensitivities. Mixing lavender oil with equal parts frankincense oil will help boost skin health.

SUPER 7 RX USES
LEMON

1. Promotes Lymphatic Drainage

Lemon oil is beneficial for improving blood flow and reducing swelling in lymph nodes. Apply 1 to 2 drops topically directly to your lymph nodes or diffuse it.

2. Helps Clear Mucus and Phlegm

Lemon oil helps to relieve congestion and eliminate mucus. It can also slow a runny nose and reduce the symptoms of allergies. Inhale lemon oil directly from the bottle or apply it topically, mixed with a carrier oil, to your chest and nose.

3. May Improve Mood

Help lift mood, improve concentration, fight depression and combat addiction by diffusing lemon essential oil, or apply it topically to your wrists and chest.

4. Assists in Gallbladder Health and Gallstone Removal

To help pass painful gallstones, mix 1 quart of sauerkraut juice, 1 quart of tomato juice, 10 drops of lemon oil and 10 drops of peppermint oil. Divide the mixture into two jars. Drink one jar the first morning, and the second jar the following morning.

5. Boosts the Immune System

Lemon essential oil has anti-bacterial properties, and it helps the body get rid of toxins that could lead to illness. Research shows that lemon oil protects the body against human pathogens such as E. coli and salmonella. To boost the immune system, take it internally.

6. Proves Effective for Cleaning Multiple Surfaces

Disinfect and degrease your home, car or office with lemon oil. Add it to a spray bottle of water to clean tables, countertops and other surfaces. Lemon oil also makes a great furniture polish; simply add a few drops to olive oil to clean, protect and shine wood.

7. Lessens Allergy Symptoms

Lemon oil can help to combat seasonal allergies and asthma attacks. It works as a natural antihistamine, relieves excess mucus and cools down inflammation. Take 1 to 2 drops internally mixed with equal parts of peppermint and lavender for allergy relief.

SUPER 7 RX USES
LEMONGRASS

1. Repels Bugs

Lemongrass oil is a natural repellant with a mild smell. Add 10 to 15 drops to water and use the mixture as bug spray, or diffuse it to repel insects. Lemongrass oil can also be used to help repel fleas by adding 5 drops of the oil to water and applying it to the pet's coat.

2. Promotes Skin Health

Lemongrass oil's antiseptic and astringent properties make it perfect for getting even and glowing skin. Add lemongrass oil to shampoos, conditioners, deodorants, soaps and lotions.

3. Acts as a Natural Deodorizer

Use lemongrass oil as a natural and safe air freshener or deodorizer. Add 5 to 10 drops of lemongrass oil to water and use it as a mist, or diffuse it. You can customize the fragrance by adding lavender or peppermint oil.

4. Treats Gastric Ulcers

Lemongrass has been known for centuries as a treatment for stomach distress, gastritis and gastric ulcers. Add lemongrass oil or infused lemongrass water to tea, soup or a smoothie to treat stomach pains, nausea and diarrhea.

5. Acts as a Fever Reducer

Consuming lemongrass oil or a lemongrass infusion has been known to reduce fevers. Lab studies have shown that a lemongrass infusion is effective in relieving feverish symptoms.

6. Lowers Cholesterol

Consumption of lemongrass oil has been shown to sustain healthy levels of triglycerides and reduce LDL cholesterol in the body. To lower cholesterol levels, take 1 to 2 drops of lemongrass oil internally in a capsule or glass of water.

7. Treats Candida/Yeast Infections

Lemongrass oil can decrease the severity of yeast infections. Take 1 to 2 drops internally.

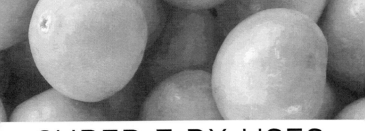

SUPER 7 RX USES
LIME

1. Eases a Sore Throat

Lime oil's powerful anti-bacterial, antiseptic and anti-viral properties help protect the body against infections that may lead to a sore throat. Take 1 to 2 drops internally by placing the oil under your tongue, or apply 2 to 4 drops topically, along with peppermint, on your throat.

2. Cleanses Water

Because it can help kill bacteria that cause diarrhea, food poisoning, cholera and typhoid, lime oil is an excellent addition to help cleanse drinking water. It also helps treat internal and external bacterial infections. Add a few drops to 8 ounces of water before consuming.

3. Encourages Lymphatic Drainage

Lime oil helps remove wastes and toxins from your body—improving immunity against pathogens. To support lymphatic flow, mix equal parts of lime oil, geranium oil and rosemary oil with coconut oil. Apply directly to your lymphatic pathways.

4. Aids Gallbladder Function and Fat Digestion

Lime oil can help clear a congested gallbladder. Mix lime oil, lemon oil and rosemary oil with a carrier oil. Add it to a compress or bath water, or massage it over your gallbladder.

5. Lifts Mood and Promotes Balance

Lime oil is stimulating and invigorating; it helps reduce anxiety and stress. Add 5 to 10 drops of lime oil to a warm-water bath, or apply it topically to your wrists, temples, abdomen, the back of your neck and the soles of your feet.

6. Repels Insects

Lime oil repels insects such as mosquitoes and ants. It can even be used to repel head lice. As a natural bug repellant, add 5 to 10 drops to a spray bottle filled with water and spray on your clothes, skin and furniture. To kill head lice, combine 5 to 10 drops of lime oil with equal parts of tea tree oil and coconut oil and massage into your hair for 10 minutes before rinsing.

7. Fights Acne and Skin Conditions

Because of its anti-bacterial and antiseptic properties, lime oil can be used on the skin to help prevent acne and skin issues. Dilute it with coconut oil or jojoba oil, and apply it to the area of concern twice daily.

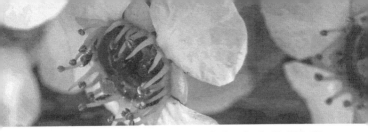

SUPER 7 RX USES
MANUKA

1. **Serves as a Remedy for Eczema, Acne and Psoriasis**

The anti-inflammatory properties of manuka oil may improve red, dry and flaking skin and conditions such as eczema, psoriasis, acne, dermatitis and cracked heels. Make a soothing cream by mixing manuka oil with shea butter for body care and honey to address acne.

2. **Calms Allergy Symptoms**

For anyone who suffers from allergic reactions to dust, pollen or pet hair, manuka oil can be used to help calm those reactions. Apply manuka oil to any area of your skin that reacts to an allergen, or diffuse 6 to 8 drops for allergy relief.

3. **Helps Heal Scars and Reduce Age Spots**

Manuka has cicatrisant properties, meaning that using it is an effective way to promote the healing of damaged skin and scarring. It can also aid in the growth and regeneration of new cells while protecting wounds from infection. Add a few drops to any face or body lotion.

4. Aids in Relaxation and Sleep

Manuka has the ability to combat stress and anxiety due to its remarkable calming and soothing effects on the heart and mind. To help relax your mind, diffuse manuka at home, at the office or by your bed to promote a good night's sleep.

5. Serves as a Natural Remedy for Athlete's Foot

Manuka oil can help eliminate a variety of fungi and bacteria that thrive on the feet and toes. Create a foot soak by adding 6 drops of manuka oil to warm water and soaking your feet for 20 minutes each day.

6. Calms Respiratory Conditions

Inhaling manuka oil can help treat respiratory conditions, such as sinus congestion, asthma and cold and flu symptoms. Diffuse it, or add 6 to 8 drops to boiling water and breathe in its vapors for 5 minutes.

7. Promotes Oral Health

Manuka has been clinically demonstrated as a potential remedy for the bacteria responsible for gum and tooth disease.[8]

---

8. Takarada, K., Kimizuka, R., Takahashi, N., Honma, K., Okuda, K., Kato, T. (2004, February). A comparison of the antibacterial efficacies of essential oils against oral pathogens. *Oral Microbiol Immunol.* Retrieved from http://www.ncbi.nlm.nih.gov/pubmed/14678476

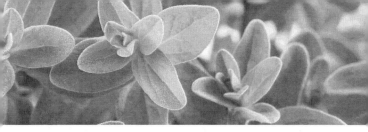

SUPER 7 RX USES
MARJORAM

1. Prevents and Improves Gastric Ulcers

Marjoram oil has shown an ability to prevent and help gastric ulcers. Take 1 to 2 drops of marjoram oil internally until symptoms subside. The herb can also be taken as a tea or supplement.

2. Helps Alleviate Headaches, Neck Pain and Back Pain

Marjoram oil can help reduce the pain that often comes with tension headaches and neck pain. Marjoram relaxes tense muscles and improves circulation, which can have pain-reducing effects for conditions caused by tight muscles. Apply it topically to areas of pain.

3. Relieves Muscle Pain and Spasms

Marjoram oil works to relieve muscle tension and pain due to overexertion. It may also alleviate some of the pain associated with the common cold, fevers, inflammation and toothaches. Dilute 3 to 5 drops and apply it topically to the area of concern twice daily.

4. Helps Prevent Infections

Due to its anti-bacterial, antiseptic and anti-viral properties, marjoram oil may help prevent infections and ailments such as the common cold, influenza, measles, mumps and cold sores. Dilute 2 to 5 drops and apply it topically twice daily.

5. Aids in Stress and Anxiety Relief

Marjoram oil has sedative properties and works to help create a calming and peaceful feeling. Diffuse marjoram oil or inhale it directly from the bottle. For topical use, dilute and apply it to the back of your neck and wrists.

6. Helps with Stomach Cramps and Flatulence

Marjoram oil helps to treat constipation, flatulence and colic by relaxing the digestive system with its sedative properties. Take it internally by placing 1 drop under your tongue, or dilute and apply it topically to your abdomen and lower back.

7. May Regulate Blood Pressure

Marjoram oil has the ability to widen and relax the blood vessels, which may ease the flow of blood and reduce high blood pressure. Take it internally by placing it under your tongue, or dilute and apply it topically over your heart.

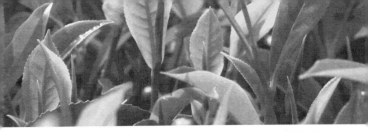

SUPER 7 RX USES
MELALEUCA

1. **Treats Acne**

Tea tree oil is considered one of the most effective home treatments for acne. It is reportedly just as effective as benzoyl peroxide but without the associated negative side effects that many people experience. Create a gentle and effective face wash by mixing 5 drops of tea tree oil with 2 teaspoons of raw honey.

2. **Helps with Dandruff**

Tea tree oil soothes dry, flaking skin and can be used as a natural treatment for head lice. Add 5 drops of tea tree oil to shampoo or conditioner, or make a natural shampoo by combining 5 to 10 drops of tea tree oil with aloe vera gel, coconut milk and lavender oil.

3. **Disinfects the Home**

Tea tree oil has powerful anti-microbial properties, allowing it to fight bad bacteria in the home. Combine tea tree oil with water, vinegar and lemon essential oil, and add it to a spray bottle to use on countertops, kitchen appliances, showers, toilets and sinks.

4. Helps Treat Psoriasis and Eczema

Use tea tree oil to relieve skin inflammation associated with conditions such as psoriasis and eczema. Make an anti-inflammatory and soothing lotion by combining 5 drops of tea tree oil, 5 drops of lavender oil and 1 teaspoon of coconut oil. Apply it topically twice daily.

5. May Remedy Toenail Fungus and Ringworm

Because of its ability to kill fungi, tea tree oil is a great choice to use on toenail fungus, athlete's foot and ringworm. Apply it topically to the affected area. For stubborn fungi, mix tea tree with oregano oil.

6. Acts as a Natural Deodorant

Because of its anti-microbial properties, tea tree oil can destroy the bacteria on the skin that causes body odor. Combine 5 drops of tea tree oil with 1 teaspoon each of coconut oil and baking soda. Apply the mixture to your armpits or even in your shoes or sports gear.

7. Cleans Infections and Cuts

The antiseptic and anti-bacterial properties of tea tree oil make it a natural treatment for cuts, wounds, burns and skin infections or irritations. Combine 2 drops of tea tree oil with 2 drops of lavender oil, and apply it directly to the area of concern.

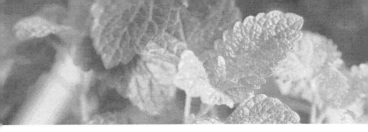

SUPER 7 RX USES
MELISSA

1. **May Help Prevent Dementia**

Melissa is probably the most studied of the essential oils for its affect on people with Alzheimer's disease, and it is very likely one of the most effective. Diffuse it daily to potentially prevent the onset of dementia.

2. **Treats Eczema**

Melissa oil is used for treating eczema and acne, as it contains anti-bacterial and anti-fungal properties. Use 5 drops per ounce of carrier oil, especially for use on the face. Alternatively, you can add it to moisturizer or a spray bottle with water and spritz on your face.

3. **Treats Cold Sores and Herpes**

Melissa is often the herb of choice for treating cold sores, as it is effective at fighting viruses in the herpes virus family. Apply 2 to 3 diluted drops topically to the area of concern.

4. May Help Improve Hypoglycemia

Studies suggest that melissa oil is an efficient hypoglycaemic agent, probably due to enhanced glucose uptake and metabolism in the liver as well as adipose tissue and the inhibition of gluconeogenesis in the liver. Take a few drops internally to promote healthy glucose levels.

5. Can Relieve Feelings of Depression and Anxiety

Melissa essential oil has antidepressant and sedative properties, and it may create a feeling of peace and warmth. It can promote emotional balance and has uplifting compounds. Diffuse or apply it topically to your wrists, ears and the back of your neck.

6. May Reduce Vertigo and Nervousness

Melissa serves as a tonic and helps the body avoid nervous disorders. Apply 2 to 3 drops topically to your ears or the back of your neck to alleviate nervousness, nausea, vomiting and dizziness. It can also be taken internally by adding 1 drop to water or tea.

7. Promotes Healthy Blood Pressure

Melissa oil has the power to reduce blood pressure levels because of its hypotensive properties. To help relieve hypertension, apply it topically to your chest or the back of your neck, or take 1 to 2 drops internally.

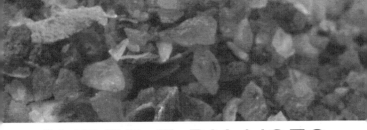

SUPER 7 RX USES
MYRRH

1. Acts as an Anti-inflammatory

Myrrh has healing, anti-bacterial, anti-fungal and anti-inflammatory properties that may reduce swelling and treat infections. Add 2 to 3 drops of myrrh oil to a cold compress and apply it directly to the infected or inflamed area.

2. Promotes Awareness During Prayer and Meditation

Because of its significance in the Bible, using myrrh is ideal during prayer and meditation. Diffuse it to help promote awareness and connect with God during meditation, and anoint others with the oil.

3. Helps Treats Vaginal and Oral Yeast

To treat Candida overgrowth, take 1 drop of myrrh oil internally, or dilute 2 to 3 drops with equal parts of a carrier oil and apply it topically to affected areas. For oral thrush, add 1 to 2 drops to natural mouthwash and gargle several times a day.

4. May Alleviate Gum Disease and Mouth Infections

Myrrh oil may help to relieve inflammation of the mouth and gums caused by diseases such as gingivitis and mouth ulcers. Add to mouthwash or toothpaste to help prevent gum disease and mouth infections.

5. Fights Parasites and Fungal Infections

Myrrh is a natural treatment for parasites, and it can also help to reduce fungal infections such as athlete's foot or ringworm. To fight infection, take 1 to 2 drops internally with water or in a capsule, or apply it directly to the fungal infection site.

6. Displays Cancer-Fighting Qualities

Myrrh is being studied for its potential anti-cancer benefits. Apply it directly to a skin cancer site twice daily. Myrrh oil is also an astringent, so it strengthens the body's cells, helps to stop bleeding and may prevent hair loss by strengthening hair roots.

7. Treats Wounds and Ulcers

Myrrh oil has the power to increase the function of white blood cells, which are critical for wound healing. It can decrease the incidence of ulcers and improve their healing time. Apply 2 to 3 drops, diluted with a carrier oil, to the affected area twice daily.

SUPER 7 RX USES
ORANGE

1. Provides Immune System Support

Orange oil has virus- and bacteria-fighting abilities. To boost the immune system and fight free radical damage, take 1 to 2 drops of orange oil internally. Place it under your tongue or add it to a glass of water or your favorite beverage.

2. Displays Cancer-Fighting Properties

The anti-cancer activity of orange oil is largely due to the presence of limonene. There are now over 200 research articles on limonene, supporting its effective chemo-preventive agents against cancer cells. Put 1 to 2 drops of orange oil into your favorite tea, juice or sparkling water.

3. Encourages Lymphatic Drainage

Orange oil may stimulate the lymphatic system, liver, kidneys and bladder—drawing out toxins, excess sodium and waste from the digestive tract. Dilute 2 to 4 drops of orange oil with coconut oil and gently rub it onto your lymph nodes, chest and lymphatic pathways.

4. Fights Anxiety

Orange essential oil is an anxiety-reducing oil thanks to its calming properties. Diffusing orange oil, adding some to your body wash or inhaling it directly may fight anxiety and lower stress levels.

5. Improves Mood

Orange oil has a direct effect on the brain's olfactory system that quickly evokes emotional responses—lifting moods and promoting relaxation. Diffuse orange oil or apply it topically.

6. Boosts Digestion

As an anti-inflammatory agent, relaxant and circulation-enhancer, orange oil promotes better digestion and may help ease cramps or constipation. Apply 2 to 3 drops to your abdominal area to boost digestion. To improve detoxification, take 1 to 2 drops internally; this encourages an increase in urine production and may prevent bloating.

7. Serves as a Natural Household Cleaner

Orange oil has a fresh and citrusy smell, and it has the power to fight bacteria and microorganisms in your home. Add orange oil to a spray bottle filled with water and use it on countertops, appliances, showers, toilets and sinks.

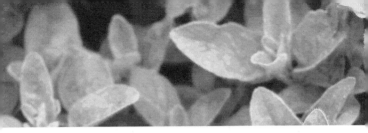

SUPER 7 RX USES
OREGANO

1. Acts as a Natural Antibiotic

Oregano oil has anti-bacterial properties that are powerful enough to kill different types of bad bacteria, including E. Coli. It can prevent bacterial overgrowth and colonization in the large intestine, and it helps protect the body from toxicity. Dilute it with a carrier oil and apply it topically to the soles of your feet or take it internally for 10 days at a time and then cycle off.

2. Battles Candida and Fungal Overgrowth

Oil of oregano can be used to treat fungi and yeast such as candida. Oregano can also treat toenail fungus when used topically. For internal use, take 2 to 4 drops twice daily for up to 10 days.

3. Helps Fight Pneumonia and Bronchitis

Oregano oil can help prevent or fight pneumonia, bronchitis and other types of bacterial infections. For external infections, apply 2 to 3 diluted drops to the affected area. To prevent internal bacterial overgrowth, ingest 2 to 4 drops twice daily for up to 10 days.

4. Proves Effective Against MRSA and Staph Infection

Oregano is the oil of choice for acute MRSA and other staph infections. Add 3 drops of oregano oil to a capsule or to the food or beverage of your choice along with a carrier oil; take it twice daily for up to 10 days.

5. Fights Intestinal Worms and Parasites

Because oregano oil has anti-parasitic and anti-viral properties, it can be used internally to combat parasitic infections. Take oregano oil internally for up to 10 days.

6. Helps Removes Warts

One of the more common uses of oregano oil is its ability to safely diminish and possibly remove warts. When using oregano oil for removing warts, make sure to dilute it with another oil or mix it with clay.

7. Cleanses Mold From the Home

Oregano is effective at eradicating mold growth around your home. Add 5 to 7 drops to a homemade cleaning solution along with tea tree oil and lavender.

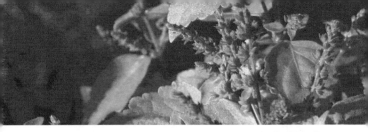

SUPER 7 RX USES
PATCHOULI

1. Helps Ease Anxiety and Fight Depression

Patchouli oil has antidepressant properties; when used aromatically, it encourages the release of serotonin and dopamine, which help to ease feelings of anger, anxiety and anxiousness. Diffuse 5 drops of patchouli oil, or add 5 to 10 drops to a warm-water bath.

2. May Reduce Inflammation

Patchouli oil has anti-phlogistic properties, meaning it has the power to soothe inflammation in the body. Patchouli oil can address internal inflammation and conditions such as arthritis and gout. Rub 3 to 5 drops onto your feet, stomach, lower back and any other inflamed area.

3. Fights Infections

With antiseptic properties, patchouli oil can protect wounds or sores from becoming infected. It can also fight athlete's foot or other fungal infections. To fight infections, apply patchouli oil directly on the affected area, or add it to a warm-water bath.

4. May Help Erectile Dysfunction

Patchouli oil has the power to increase libido. It also serves as a natural supplement for helping with impotency and erectile dysfunction. Diffuse 5 drops of patchouli oil, or apply 1 to 3 drops topically to your temples, the back of your neck and the soles of your feet.

5. Strengthens Hair and Skin

Patchouli oil may prevent hair loss and regenerate new skin cells. For hair, massage it into your scalp or add it to conditioner. For your skin, dilute patchouli oil with equal parts of coconut or jojoba oil and apply it topically, or add it to face wash or lotion.

6. Repels Insects

Patchouli oil repels mosquitoes, fleas, ants, lice, moths and flies. Add 5 to 10 drops to a spray bottle filled with water and spray on your clothes, skin, sheets or furniture.

7. Acts as a Natural Deodorant

Patchouli oil has a sweet, musky and spicy aroma; it can be used to mask body odor. It also makes a great home deodorizer. Apply it under your arms, or add it to your favorite lotion.

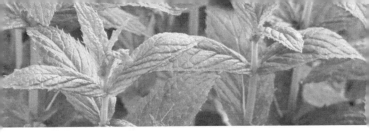

SUPER 7 RX USES
PEPPERMINT

1. **Helps Relieve Muscle Pain**

Peppermint oil may help reduce pain and relax muscles. It is especially helpful in soothing an aching back, sore muscles and tension headaches. Dilute 2 to 4 drops and apply it topically to the area of concern.

2. Soothes Respiratory Conditions

Peppermint oil acts as an expectorant and may relieve some symptoms of a respiratory illness. Dilute 2 to 4 drops and apply it topically to your chest and the back of your neck. Alternatively, you can add 10 drops to boiling water, put a towel over your head and breathe in the aroma for 5 minutes.

3. Boosts Energy

Because peppermint is invigorating and stimulating, it can help fight chronic fatigue and improve concentration. Diffuse it, or apply it to your temples, wrists and the back of your neck. It can also be inhaled directly for a quick energy boost.

4. Helps Reduce Allergy Symptoms

Peppermint helps relax the muscles in the nasal passages and clear out mucus and pollen during allergy season. Diffuse 5 drops, inhale it directly from the bottle or dilute 2 to 3 drops and apply it topically to your forehead, neck and chest.

5. Aids in Headache Relief

Peppermint oil may improve circulation, soothe the gut and relax tense muscles. It can also help clear your nasal passages when you're suffering from a sinus headache. Apply it to your forehead and temples for pain relief.

6. Eases Digestive Conditions

Peppermint oil helps to relax the muscles in the intestines and reduce bloating, gas and nausea. It may also serve as a natural remedy for irritable bowel syndrome. Diffuse it, apply it topically to your abdomen, or take 1 to 2 drops internally.

7. Freshens Breath and Fights Cavities

Peppermint oil has anti-microbial properties that will freshen breath and may kill bacteria that lead to cavities and gum disease. Add 1 drop to toothpaste or mouthwash, or place the oil under your tongue before drinking a glass of water.

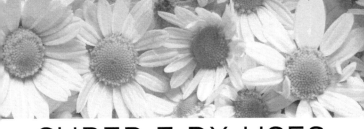

SUPER 7 RX USES
ROMAN CHAMOMILE

1. Helps Fight Anxiety and Depression

Roman chamomile fights stress and promotes relaxation. Inhaling Roman chamomile is a natural remedy for anxiety; the fragrance is carried directly to the brain and serves as an emotional trigger. Diffuse 5 drops, or inhale it directly from the bottle.

2. May Improve Digestion and Leaky Gut

Roman chamomile oil contains anodyne compounds that are antispasmodic and can be used to remedy various gastrointestinal disturbances, from gas to leaky gut to acid reflux. Use in low doses for children with colic and diarrhea. Apply 2-4 drops topically to the abdomen.

3. Encourages Restful Sleep

The relaxing properties of Roman chamomile promotes healthy sleep and fights insomnia. Diffuse next to bed, rub onto temples or inhale directly from the bottle.

4. Calms and Soothes Children

For centuries, mothers have used

Roman chamomile to calm crying children, reduce fevers, eliminate earaches and soothe upset stomachs. It even helps children with ADD/ADHD. Either diffuse it or apply it topically.

5. Boosts Skin Health

Roman chamomile promotes smooth, healthy skin because of its anti-inflammatory and anti-bacterial properties. Use to fight acne, various skin conditions and signs of aging. Add 2 to 3 drops to a cotton ball and apply it to the area of concern, or add 5 drops to a face wash.

6. Promotes Heart Health

Roman chamomile provides cardiovascular protection because of its high levels of flavonoids. It may lower blood pressure and relax the heart. Apply 2 to 4 drops topically over your heart, or take it internally by placing it under your tongue.

7. Eases Nausea

Because of its relaxing properties, Roman chamomile can relieve nausea associated with pregnancy or motion sickness. Inhale directly from the bottle, or combine it with ginger, peppermint and lavender oil and diffuse. It can also be used topically on your temples for nausea.

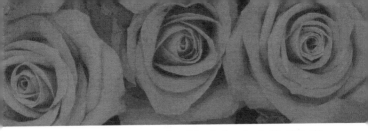

SUPER 7 RX USES
ROSE

1. Helps Fight Depression

Rose essential oil has sedative properties that can create a relaxing and peaceful feeling. Combine rose oil with lavender oil and diffuse it, or apply 1 to 2 drops topically to your wrists and the back of your neck.

2. Can Boost Libido

Because it acts as an anti-anxiety agent, rose essential oil can help treat sexual dysfunction related to feelings of anxiety and stress. It helps to balance hormones and can increase sex drive. Diffuse it, or apply 2 to 3 drops topically to your neck and chest.

3. Promotes Skin Health

The anti-microbial properties of rose oil make it a powerful treatment for skin conditions, including acne. It can also help prevent scarring, minimize the look of wrinkles and alleviate poison ivy rashes. Apply it topically or add to face wash, body wash or lotion.

4. Aids Digestion

Because of the relaxing properties present in rose essential oil, it can help improve digestive issues that are related to stress and anxiety. Apply 2 to 3 drops topically to your abdomen to help ease stomachaches.

5. Helps with PMS and Menstrual Symptoms

Due to its anti-spasmodic properties, rose essential oil may relieve cramps associated with PMS and menstruation. It also fights feelings of moodiness and anxiety. Diffuse it, or apply it topically to your abdomen.

6. May Relieve Seizures

The anti-spasmodic and sedative properties of rose oil can help people who experience seizures. Diffuse it, or apply it topically to your wrists and the back of your neck.

7. Serves as a Fragrant Perfume

The sweet, inviting smell of rose essential oil serves as a superior alternative to synthetic perfumes. Simply dab 1 to 2 drops behind your ears or on your wrists. A little goes a long way!

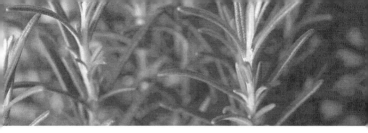

SUPER 7 RX USES
ROSEMARY

1. Increases Hair Growth

Rosemary essential oil stimulates hair growth and can help prevent baldness, slow graying and treat dandruff or dry scalp. Apply 3 to 5 drops to your scalp, rub it in and allow the oil to sit for 5 minutes before rinsing, or add 5 to 10 drops to shampoo or conditioner.

2. May Improve Memory

Studies show that rosemary oil improves cognitive performance, increases alertness and enhances overall quality of memory. Add it to a diffuser, or apply it topically under your nose or across your forehead.

3. Acts as a Natural Diabetes Remedy

Over time, incorporating rosemary oil into your daily routine can help to supplement and assist in the body's balance and regulation of hormones and blood sugar levels. Take 1 to 2 drops in a glass of water.

4. Helps Reduce Pain

Because of rosemary oil's anti-inflammatory properties, it has the power to reduce joint and muscle pain. Mix 2 drops of rosemary oil, 2 drops of peppermint oil and 1 teaspoon of coconut oil and rub it onto sore muscles and painful joints.

5. Promotes Liver Detox and Gallbladder Function

Using rosemary oil topically can enhance the performance of the bile-producing gallbladder and help to prevent toxin buildup in the body. Mix 3 drops of rosemary oil with ¼ teaspoon of coconut oil and rub it over your gallbladder area twice daily.

6. Aids in Detoxifying the Body

Rosemary oil boosts nutrient absorption and helps to reverse or prevent toxic overload. Take it internally, or apply 2 to 3 drops to your abdomen to detoxify your body.

7. Fights Respiratory Issues

Rosemary oil works as an expectorant—reducing mucus and relieving some of the symptoms of bronchitis, cold and other respiratory infections. Apply it topically to your chest, or diffuse it, to thin and expel mucus.

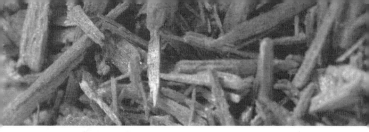

SUPER 7 RX USES
SANDALWOOD

1. **Promotes Mental Clarity and Memory**

Sandalwood essential oil is frequently used in meditation and prayer because of its ability to promote mental clarity. May help Alzheimer's disease sufferers. Diffuse or apply 2 to 3 drops topically to your wrists and under your nose.

2. **Can Boost Low Testosterone**

For men with low testosterone, adding a few drops of sandalwood oil to homemade deodorant or homemade lotion is a great way to get some extra health benefits by promoting hormone balance.

3. **Acts as an Aphrodisiac**

Sandalwood oil is a natural anti-inflammatory agent that helps reduce swelling and bloating. Santalol, an active ingredient in sandalwood oil, can decrease cytokines (inflammation markers in the body). Apply 3 to 5 drops to the area of concern.

4. May Reduce Inflammation

Sandalwood oil is a natural anti-inflammatory agent that will help reduce swelling and bloating. Santalol, an active ingredient in sandalwood oil, can decrease cytokines (inflammation markers in the body). Apply 3 to 5 drops to the area of concern.

5. Supports Healthy Blood Pressure

Studies have found that sandalwood oil may decrease systolic blood pressure when applied directly to the skin. This can be due to its calming and sedative properties. Apply it topically to your chest, wrists and the back of your neck.

6. Inhibits Tumor Growth

Studies suggest that sandalwood oil has anti-cancer and chemo-protective effects when used internally. It may inhibit the growth of cancer cells and can be used as a natural anti-cancer agent. Take 1 to 2 drops of sandalwood oil internally.

7. Acts as a Natural Deodorant and Cologne

With its rich, woodsy aroma, sandalwood makes an excellent deodorant and cologne. To make your own deodorant, mix 10 drops of sandalwood, 4 tablespoons of coconut oil, 4 tablespoons of baking soda and 4 tablespoons of cornstarch. Store in the fridge.

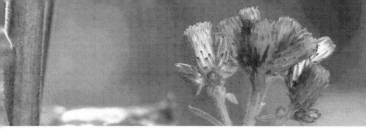

SUPER 7 RX USES
SPIKENARD

1. **Displays Antibiotic Properties**

When applied topically to wounds, spikenard can fight
bacteria. Inside the body, spikenard helps treat bacterial
infections in the kidneys, bladder and urethra. Apply 3
to 5 drops topically to the area of concern, or take 1 to 2
drops internally for infection and diffuse.

2. **Can Reduce Inflammation**

Spikenard oil relieves inflammation, which is at the
root of many conditions and diseases such as asthma,
arthritis, Crohn's disease, Alzheimer's disease, cancer,
cardiovascular disease, diabetes, high blood pressure,
high cholesterol and Parkinson's disease. Apply 3 to 5
drops topically twice daily, diffuse the oil or take 1 drop
internally each day.

3. **Helps Reduce Stress and Anxiety**

Spikenard oil is relaxing and soothing for the skin and
mind; it's often used as a sedative and calming agent.
Diffuse spikenard oil or apply it topically.

4. Boosts the Immune System

Spikenard oil is an immune system booster because it calms the body, enabling it to function properly. To boost your immune system, diffuse spikenard or apply it topically to the soles of your feet or the back of your neck.

5. Promotes Hair Growth

Spikenard oil is known for promoting hair growth, helping to retain its natural color and slowing down the process of graying. Add 5 to 10 drops to a bottle of shampoo or conditioner, or combine 5 drops of spikenard oil with 1 teaspoon of coconut oil and massage the mixture into your scalp; let it sit for 5 minutes before rinsing.

6. Treats Insomnia

Spikenard's sedative and relaxing properties can be helpful to those with insomnia or sleep deprivation. Diffuse or apply 2 to 3 drops topically to your temples and the back of your neck.

7. Helps with Constipation

Spikenard oil is a natural laxative, and it stimulates the digestive system, helping to naturally relieve constipation. Apply spikenard oil onto your stomach and the soles of your feet.

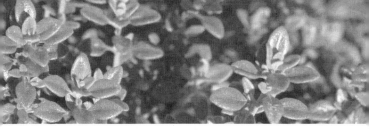

SUPER 7 RX USES
THYME

1. Improves Respiratory Conditions

Thyme oil is anti-bacterial, anti-fungal, spasmolytic and expectorant, so it helps quell bronchitis and a spasmodic cough. Diffuse it, apply it topically to your chest and neck, take 1 to 2 drops internally or add 5 to 7 drops of thyme oil to boiling water and breathe in the steam.

2. Battles Bacteria and Parasites

Thyme oil helps treat intestinal infections and bacterial infections in the genitals and urethra. It's useful in treating bacteria that build up in the respiratory system. Apply 2 to 4 drops directly to the affected area, or take 1 drop internally with water to battle bacteria and parasites.

3. Boosts Skin Health

Thyme oil protects the skin from harmful bacteria and fungal infections, so it can treat acne, wounds, cuts, rashes and scars. A powerful antioxidant, it can help slow the aging process as well. Apply 2 to 4 drops of thyme oil topically to the area of concern.

4. Calms Inflammatory Bowel Diseases (IBD)

Thyme can help calm IBD, Crohn's disease and colitis. Mix 1 drop each of thyme, Roman chamomile, peppermint, ginger and frankincense with a teaspoon of coconut oil. Consume this mixture with breakfast and again just before dinner until your symptoms subside, and then continue taking it twice daily for another week.

5. Serves as Insect Repellent

Thyme oil helps keep away pests and parasites that feed on the body, such as mosquitoes, fleas, lice and bed bugs. Apply it topically or diffuse it. A few drops of thyme oil placed in the closet or kitchen can also repel moths and beetles.

6. Promotes Healthy Hormone Balance

With progesterone-balancing effects, thyme oil may also relieve symptoms of menopause, including mood swings, hot flashes and insomnia. Diffuse it, or apply it to the back of your neck, on your wrists and on the soles of your feet.

7. Fights Uterine Fibroids

Uterine fibroids are caused by high levels of estrogen and low levels of progesterone. To help break them up, rub 2 drops each of thyme, clary sage and frankincense oils over your lower abdomen twice daily.

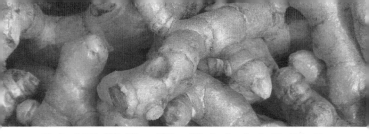

SUPER 7 RX USES
TURMERIC

1. Helps Relieve Arthritis and Joint Pain

Turmeric contains the active ingredient curcumin, which is an antioxidant that demonstrates anti-inflammatory properties in conditions such as arthritis, muscle sprains and other injuries. Add a few drops directly to the source of pain.

2. Serves as a Digestive Aid

Turmeric may help reduce symptoms of digestive conditions such as irritable bowel syndrome (IBS). Add 1 drop to your favorite tea for a spicy and beneficial kick to your beverage. Also apply it topically to your abdomen with a carrier oil.

3. Displays Promising Anti-Cancer Properties

Turmerone and curcumin in turmeric oil both displayed the ability to fight colon cancer in animal models, which may make it an effective supplement during cancer treatment. Take 1 drop internally in the morning and evening, mixed in your food or beverage. You can also mix it with a culinary carrier and consume this mixture in a capsule.

4. Fights Neurologic Diseases

Turmeric oil's aromatic turmerone is believed to be a promising way to support the regeneration necessary to improve neurologic diseases such as Parkinson's disease, Alzheimer's disease, spinal cord injury and stroke. Diffuse it, apply it topically or take it internally.

5. Relieves Depression and Anxiety

Turmeric essential oil is considered to be a strong relaxant and balancer, and studies show that it can help fight against two extremely common mood disorders, depression and anxiety. Diffuse it throughout the day to improve mood and encourage positive feelings.

6. May Help with Epilepsy

The anti-convulsant properties of turmeric oil may reduce or prevent some seizures. To aid in the prevention of seizures, take 1 to 2 drops internally or regularly drink hot turmeric tea.

7. Promotes Liver Detox

Studies have shown that turmeric is liver-protective, which is partly due to turmeric's anti-inflammatory activity. To encourage liver detoxification and help improve liver health, take it internally or apply it topically.

SUPER 7 RX USES
VETIVER

1. Helps Fight Insomnia

Vetiver is calming and relaxing, and is therefore ideal for those suffering from insomnia. Diffuse it next to your bed, inhale it directly or add a few drops to a warm bath just before bedtime.

2. Serves as a Study Aid

Vetiver inspires a harmonious state while promoting deep concentration. Diffuse vetiver oil while studying for exams or working late hours to promote clear thinking and increased concentration.

3. Fights Aging and Free Radical Damage

Vetiver oil has a strong free radical scavenging activity that helps to slow the aging process, promote healthy and glowing skin, reduce the risk of cancer and boost detoxification. Diffuse it, or apply it topically.

4. Promotes Scar Healing

Vetiver oil is a cicatrisant, meaning it heals scars by promoting the regeneration of skin and tissue. By rejuvenating the skin, vetiver oil helps to remove dark spots along with acne scarring. Apply 2 to 4 drops of vetiver oil topically to the area of concern.

5. May Help People with ADD/ADHD

An important study has shown that vetiver oil is effective in children with ADHD and ADD because of its ability to relax and calm. Combine 2 drops of vetiver oil and 2 drops of lavender oil and diffuse it, or apply it topically.

6. Can Improve Nervous Tremors

Vetiver oil has been found to reduce tremors and boost the immune and nervous systems. Diffuse 5 drops or apply 2 to 3 drops topically to your wrists, the soles of your feet and the back of your neck to help reduce tremors such as those associated with Parkinson's disease.

7. Soothes Anxiety and Nervousness

Vetiver oil has been used in aromatherapy for relaxation and alleviating emotional stress, panic attacks, trauma, anxiety, insomnia, hysteria and depression. Diffuse the oil, apply it topically or add it to a warm-water bath to relieve feelings of anxiety and stress.

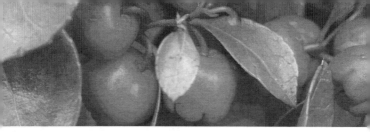

SUPER 7 RX USES
WINTERGREEN

1. **Battles Joint and Muscle Pain**

Wintergreen oil may reduce swelling and irritation that occurs around painful muscles and tissue. It can relieve sore muscles, neck pain and lower back pain. Dilute 3 to 5 drops with equal parts of a carrier oil and apply it to the areas of concern.

2. **Helps Improve Respiratory Conditions**

Wintergreen contains an aspirin-like chemical that helps to reduce pain, congestion, swelling and fever associated with common illnesses. Combine 1 to 3 drops of wintergreen with coconut oil and rub it on your chest and upper back to help open your nasal passages.

3. **Helps Fight and Prevent Infections**

Wintergreen oil helps to combat bacterial growth, viruses and fungi because of its antiseptic and disinfectant properties. Dilute it before topical application. Add 5 to 10 drops to a spray bottle filled with water and use it on your clothes, furniture and any hard surface.

4. Addresses Gout Symptoms

Wintergreen oil stimulates the organs in the urinary system and the filtration of water by the kidneys, increasing the frequency and quantity of urine. This speeds up the removal of toxins like uric acid. Combine it with coconut oil and apply it to areas of concern.

5. Promotes Skin Health

As a natural astringent and antiseptic, wintergreen is able to fight inflammation from blemishes and skin disorders like acne. Add 1 to 2 drops to a face wash or apply it to the areas of concern.

6. Combats Fatigue

Respiratory-improving wintergreen oil may increase stamina, alertness and endurance. Inhale wintergreen oil directly from the bottle before a workout, or dilute and apply it topically to your neck, chest and wrists to fight sleepiness and fatigue.

7. Serves as a DIY Mouthwash and Toothpaste

Wintergreen oil fights germs in the mouth and is able to freshen breath and prevent mouth irritants and the growth of bacteria. Add a few drops to a glass of water and gargle for 30 to 60 seconds before rinsing. Do not swallow.

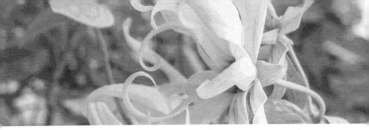

SUPER 7 RX USES
YLANG YLANG

1. **Helps Regulate Blood Pressure**

Ylang ylang supports a healthy circulatory system.
It's considered one of the most helpful essential oils
for controlling blood pressure and preventing heart
arrhythmia. Dilute it and apply 1 drop topically over your
heart, or add 2 drops to a cup of water or warm tea.

2. **Promotes Skin Health**

When applied to the skin, ylang ylang oil may help
prevent signs of aging. It may even help fight the
development of skin cancer cells, including melanoma.
Combine 2 drops with equal parts of coconut or jojoba oil
and apply it topically to the area of concern twice daily.

3. **Boosts Mood and Energy**

Acting directly on the olfactory system of the brain, inhaling
ylang ylang oil can have immediate, positive effects on
your mood and act like a mild, natural depression remedy.
Combine 3 to 5 drops with a carrier oil and massage it onto
your temples and the back of your neck.

4. Helps Balance Hormones

Ylang ylang oil helps to reduce the cramps, tension and stress associated with PMS. Combine 2 drops of ylang ylang and 2 drops of lavender, and apply the mixture topically to the back of your neck and on your lower abdomen.

5. May Lessen Frustration and Anger

Ylang ylang oil aids in releasing negative emotions, including anger, low self-esteem and jealousy. Diffuse it, or inhale it directly from the bottle to help wash away frustration.

6. Encourages Self-Confidence

Inhaling ylang ylang can have immediate, positive effects on your self-confidence. It can empower you and help you take on life's challenges with greater confidence and optimism. Inhale it directly, diffuse it or apply it to your wrists and the back of your neck.

7. Serves as a Natural Aphrodisiac

Ylang ylang has been shown to act like a natural impotence remedy and help increase the libido of both men and women. It boosts energy and creates feelings of relaxation. Diffuse it, or apply it topically to your temples, wrists or the back of your neck.

CARRIER OILS

Carrier oils are used to dilute essential oils when they are being used topically; they help to *carry* the essential oils into the skin. Many lotions and skin care products are made with carrier oils, which are vegetable oils derived from the fatty portion of the plant, like the nuts, kernels or seeds. Unlike essential oils, carrier oils do not evaporate easily and do not give off strong aromas. Unfortunately, carrier oils often have a defined shelf life and will become rancid over time.

Each carrier oil offers a different combination of nourishing properties, benefits and characteristics. Some are more aromatic than others, and the color and shelf life will differ as well. The following pages will provide you with some of the most widely used carrier oils that can be combined with essential oils in aromatherapy.

Almond

Almond oil presents a variety of health benefits: It addresses bad cholesterol, helps prevent inflammation, hydrates dry skin and supports cardiovascular health. This oil has even been presented as an alternative, renewable biofuel source. When used topically, it is known for its ability to soften and soothe inflamed skin. It absorbs into the skin fairly quickly, leaving a slight hint of oil.

Apricot Kernel

The kernels of the apricot fruit are cold-pressed to extract the beneficial oils. This oil works great as a massage oil because it is very light and soothing to the skin. In Traditional Chinese Medicine, apricot kernel oil is used to treat tumors and ulcers. It has also been used to relieve digestive issues and boost skin health.

Arnica

Arnica oil has been used for medicinal purposes since the 1500s. It contains helenalin, a potent anti-inflammatory agent, which is why arnica oil is commonly used on the skin in the form of an oil, cream, ointment, liniment or salve. This carrier oil needs to be diluted before topical use. When purchased from a store, arnica oil should already be diluted and ready for use, but make sure to read the label carefully. When applied to the skin, it helps to reduce pain caused by inflammation, while also treating bruises, aches, sprains and even arthritis flare-ups.

Argan

For generations, natives of the Argan Forest in Morocco have pressed the argan nut to extract this precious oil to use as a dietary supplement for wound healing and rash relief, and to nourish skin and hair. Argan oil is rich in vitamins A and E; it is also packed with antioxidants, omega-6 fatty acids and linoleic acid. When it is applied topically, it eases inflammation, moisturizes skin and boosts cell production.

Avocado

Avocado oil has actually received prescription drug status in France because of its proven ability to counter the negative effects of arthritis. This oil is produced from the fruit of the avocado tree. Because it is extracted from the fleshy pulp of the fruit, it is one of the few edible oils not derived from a seed. The pulp produces oil full of healthy fats, including oleic acid and essential fatty acids. Avocado oil can be used topically to hydrate dry hair and improve its texture, as well as improve skin health. It also reduces inflammation and boosts nutrient absorption.

Coconut

The coconut tree is considered the "tree of life" in much of
Southeast Asia, India, the Philippines and other tropical
locations. Today, there are over 1,500 articles demonstrating
the health benefits of coconut oil. The uses are numerous
thanks to its natural healing properties and tremendous use
as a product for natural beauty treatments and so much
more.

Evening Primrose

Primrose is a wild flower that grows in eastern and central
North America. The seeds of the flower are cold-pressed
for the extraction of their oil, which is high in essential
fatty acids. Evening primrose oil has a range of therapeutic
properties; it is known to help reduce the pain associated
with PMS and relieve skin irritations and conditions. The oil
could also be used as an anti-inflammatory agent, and it
is commonly used to relieve problems with autoimmune
diseases.

Hemp

Hemp seed is an all-natural way to jumpstart better skin
with a wave of incredible vitamins. Hemp seed oil does
not contain THC (tetrahydrocannabinol) or the other
psychoactive constituents that are present in the dried leaves
of Cannabis sativa. With generous amounts of omega fatty
acids and proteins, this oil wonderfully reinvigorates the
skin as it helps to clear away acne and eczema. Extremely
emollient and absorbent, hemp seed oil is packed with
vitamins A, B1, B2, B3, B6, C, D and E. It also has abundant
levels of anti-inflammatory and antioxidant properties. Hemp
seed oil also reduces toxins while alleviating sore muscles
and joints.

Jojoba

Jojoba oil (pronounced ho-ho-ba) is the liquid that comes from the seed of the Simmondsia chinensis plant. It is labeled as an oil, but is actually a liquid plant wax that has been used in folk medicine for a number of ailments. Because jojoba is an emollient, it soothes the skin and unclogs hair follicles. It can be combined with essential oils such as lavender or peppermint to boost skin and hair health.

Olive

Olive trees have been around for many thousands of years. With a long history dating back to ancient civilizations, olive oil is even considered to be one of the most important Bible foods. High-quality olive oil has well-researched anti-inflammatory compounds and antioxidants. It is made from the fruit of the olive tree, which is naturally high in healthy fatty acids. When used topically, olive oil reduces oxidative damage and works as an anti-microbial agent. It should be used in small amounts, as the olive fragrance could overpower the aroma of essential oils when used in high doses.

Pomegranate

Pomegranate seed oil is considered one of the Bible's powerful foods because of its powerful anti-aging benefits. The dark red color in pomegranate seed oil comes from the bioflavonoids, which protect the skin from sun damage. It has a natural sun protection factor (SPF) and can be used as a sunblock and sunscreen.

Rosehip

Rosehip oil is harvested from the seeds of rose bushes predominately grown in Chile. It contains powerful antioxidants, vitamins and essential fatty acids—making it an effective carrier oil for hydrating the skin, relieving itchiness and minimizing the appearances of dark spots, scars and fine lines. Rosehip absorbs easily, and it is non-greasy and light when applied topically.

Sea Buckthorn

Sea buckthorn berries and seeds are cold-pressed and CO_2 extracted for their oils, which are rich in essential fatty acids and contain vitamins, minerals and nutritive compounds. Sea buckthorn oil is used on the skin to reduce the signs of aging. Because of its intense color that can stain skin when used in high doses, a 1:3 dilution is recommended.

Shea Butter

Shea butter is not a carrier oil, but its natural, beneficial properties make it a lipid suitable for aromatherapy work. It is highly moisturizing, has a smooth, creamy texture and can be included in massage blends, lotions, creams and other natural skin care products. Shea butter can become gritty if not melted and then cooled properly. Once it has cooled, it does not need to be kept in the refrigerator.

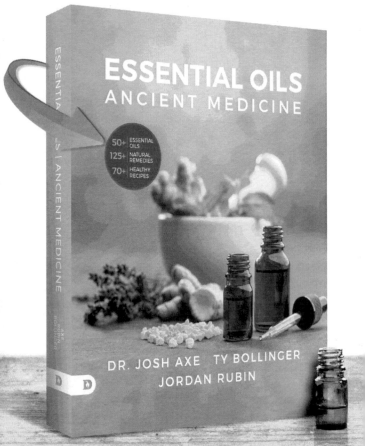